Seven LEE of Life

Anthology of Wisdom by 108 Visionaries

Compiled by

ABHISHAIK CHITRAANS
RAINU MANGTANI

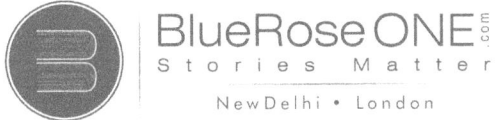

BLUEROSE PUBLISHERS
India | U.K.

Copyright © Abhishaik Chitraans 2024

All rights reserved by author. No part of this publication may be reproduced, stored in a retrieval system or transmitted in any form or by any means, electronic, mechanical, photocopying, recording or otherwise, without the prior permission of the author. Although every precaution has been taken to verify the accuracy of the information contained herein, the publisher assumes no responsibility for any errors or omissions. No liability is assumed for damages that may result from the use of information contained within.

BlueRose Publishers takes no responsibility for any damages, losses, or liabilities that may arise from the use or misuse of the information, products, or services provided in this publication.

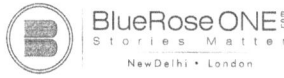

For permissions requests or inquiries regarding this publication,
please contact:

BLUEROSE PUBLISHERS
www.BlueRoseONE.com
info@bluerosepublishers.com
+91 8882 898 898
+4407342408967

ISBN: 978-93-6452-199-4

Cover Design: Sadhna Kumari
Typesetting: Pooja Sharma

First Edition: December 2024

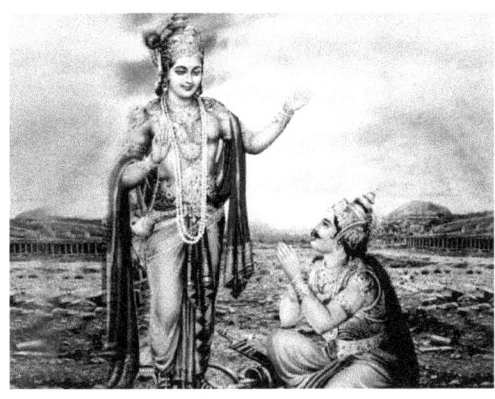

वसुदेवसुतं देवं कंसचाणूरमर्दनम्। देवकीपरमानन्दं कृष्णं वन्दे जगद्गुरूम्॥

Seven LEE of Life

[Anthology of Wisdom by 108 Visionaries]

A collection of articles showing real life's Learning, Earning, Expectation with diversity of thoughts

(108 x 7 x 3 = 2,268 points to read/ observe in one book)

Compiled by

Internationally Renowned Author Couple

Rainu Mangtani
Abhishaik Chitraans

(ईष्ट कृपा एवं गुरु आशीष)

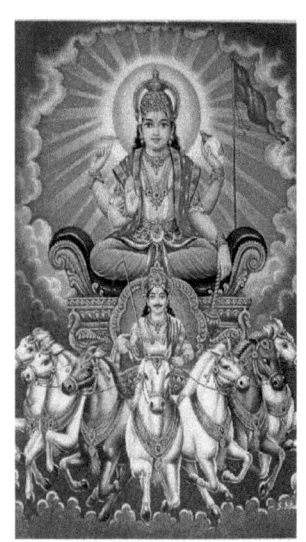

|| प्रार्थना ||

ॐ असतो मा सद्गमय

तमसो मा ज्योतिर्गमय

मृत्योर्मा अमृतं गमय

|| ॐ शान्तिः शान्तिः शान्तिः ||

Disclaimer

The content of *'Seven LEE of Life'* represents the personal insights, experiences and viewpoints. *It is a collaborative anthology reflecting diverse perspectives on Learning, Earning and Expectation of each contributing co-author.* The opinions and advice shared within this anthology are meant for educational and inspirational purposes only. Each contributor's ideas, views and recommendations are based on their unique life's experiences and insights. While every effort has been made to ensure the accuracy of the information provided, readers should use their discretion and consult professionals when necessary.

This book does not serve as professional advice and the compilers Mr. Abhishaik Chitraans and Mrs. Rainu Mangtani, along with the publisher, assume no liability for outcomes arising from the application of any ideas presented herein.

॥ ॐ ॥

Dedication

This anthology *'Seven LEE of Life'* is dedicated to all the seekers of wisdom, the dreamers of prosperity and the believers in a brighter future;

- Who believes in the power of knowledge, the dignity of honest work and the courage to dream big.

- Who strive for growth through **Learning**, find purpose through **Earning** and hold boundless **Expectation** for themselves and the world around them.

This book is dedicated to the visionaries, mentors and life-long learners, who inspire others to pursue their potential. To the individuals who redefine success by sharing wisdom and lifting those around them and to those who carry the torch of hope and resilience in their hearts.

May these pages/ collection of insights inspire, guide and empower readers to embark on their own journeys of self-discovery, success and fulfilment.

With gratitude to all 108 contributors/ co-authors, whose voices illuminate this path.

॥ ॐ ॥

Preface

In a world shaped by rapid change and boundless potential, we all seek a roadmap to success, wisdom and fulfilment. *'Seven LEE of Life'* was born from this shared pursuit—a collective journey into the realms of **Learning, Earning** and **Expectation** or *LEE*. This anthology is more than just a compilation; it's a tapestry woven from the insights, aspirations and life lessons of 108 visionaries, who each hold unique perspectives on achieving growth and purpose.

Each contributor to *'Seven LEE of Life'* brings forward their own experiences and understanding, articulating seven key points under each of the three guiding pillars. From hard-earned wisdom to innovative strategies and unyielding dreams, these reflections aim to serve as a source of inspiration, motivation and practical guidance.

Compiled by the internationally renowned author couple **Mr. Abhishaik Chitraans** and **Mrs. Rainu Mangtani,** this anthology serves as a lighthouse for anyone navigating their personal or professional journey. It is a testament to the power of shared insights and the strength found in diverse voices united by a common purpose.

May this collection open new doors of thought, encourage readers to set their sights high and fuel the desire to make meaningful contributions in their own lives and in the lives of others.

॥ ॐ ॥

Acknowledgement

Bringing *'Seven LEE of Life'* to life has been an inspiring journey, one that would not have been possible without the support and contributions of many.

First and foremost, we extend our heartfelt gratitude to the 108 remarkable and eminent co-authors, whose wisdom, passion and dedication have transformed this anthology into a beacon of insight. Each one of you has generously shared a part of your journey and your words will continue to resonate with readers seeking guidance on their paths of Learning, Earning, and Expectation.

A special thank you to the families, friends and mentors who have stood beside us and our co-authors, offering encouragement and support every step of the way. Your influence is woven into every page of this book.

At the end, we are also grateful to the entire publishing team, whose professionalism and attention to detail have brought clarity and coherence to this collective work. Your expertise has been invaluable in shaping our vision into reality. It is your thirst for growth and self-improvement that drives us to compile this anthology. May the words within *'Seven LEE of Life'* ignite a spark in you, as they did in us.

With deepest and heartiest gratitude,

Abhishaik Chitraans & Rainu Mangtani

॥ ॐ ॥

Understand 'LEE' – Learning, Earning, Expectation …

"We uncover purpose in learning, we build strength through earning and we find the courage to pursue our expected dreams"

"Learning sharpens our minds, earning fuels our journey and expectation gives life to our vision of success."

"We grow with each step in learning; we empower ourselves through earning and we unlock our potential through expectation."

[Rainu Mangtani]   **[Abhishaik Chitraans]**

ॐ भूर्भुवः स्वः तत् सवितुर्वरेण्यं भर्गो देवस्य धीमहि धियो यो नः प्रचोदयात् ॥

॥ ॐ ॥

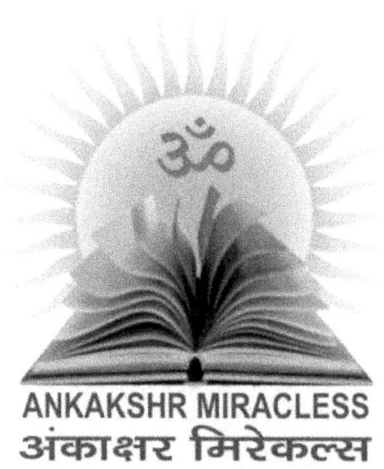

ANKAKSHR MIRACLESS
अंकाक्षर मिरेकल्स

The Institute of Occult Sciences, Spiritual Activities and Research
Regd. by Ministry of MSME, Govt. of India
ISO 9001:2015 Certified
IVAF & AAA (USA) Recognized

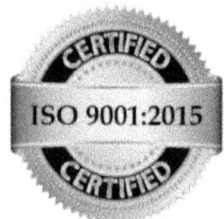 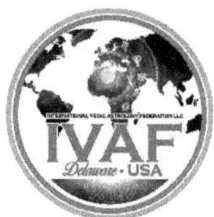

IVAF : International Vedic Astrology Federation (USA)
(An American Organization of Research)
AAA : Astrological Academic Alliances (USA)
(The World's Best International Astrology Forum

www.abhishaikchitraans.com

|| ॐ ||

Contents

Foreword by Nivedita Basu 1

Foreword by Sidhharrth S Kumaar 3

Foreword by Sneha 5

The Family of Visionary Co-authors 7

Abhishaik Chitraans (Compiler) 13

Rainu Mangtani (Compiler) 15

1. Seven LEE of Life (Compilers' Pen) 17
2. Abhilasha Bhatnagar 22
3. Acharya Madhu B Chawla 25
4. Aditya Ujjwal 27
5. Aekta Doshi 29
6. Akanksha Rebecca George 32
7. Amrit Kaur 34
8. Anita Gupta 36
9. Anu Chauhan 39
10. Anuradha Bijawara 41
11. Archana Nadella 43
12. Archana Nair 45
13. Aruna 48
14. Avneet Chaudhary 50
15. B D Surana 52
16. Baljit Jaggi 54
17. Bhavana M Patle 57
18. Binita Nandi 60
19. C P Belliappa 62
20. CA Meenaz Cyrus Surty 64
21. Deepa Jain 67
22. Deepti Sood 69
23. Divvya A Singh 71
24. Dr. A S Poovamma 74

25.	Dr. Agalya VT Raj	76
26.	Dr. Anisha Mahenrakar	78
27.	Dr. Ellakkiyaa Sankar	80
28.	Dr. Heena P	82
29.	Dr. K G Veena	85
30.	Dr. Mahima Mohit Dand	87
31.	Dr. Mehjabeen	90
32.	Dr. Navjot Kaur	93
33.	Dr. Noothan Rao	96
34.	Dr. Priti Doshi	99
35.	Dr. Priyadarshini MM	102
36.	Dr. Shalini Garg	104
37.	Giresh LD Chawda	107
38.	Harishita (Vicky Chauhan)	111
39.	Harsatvir Kaur	113
40.	Himani Bajaj	115
41.	Himani Verma	118
42.	Isha Singh	119
43.	Jiggna B Bhatt	121
44.	Kala Malpani	125
45.	Kalpana Priyadarshi	128
46.	Kanan Jolly	130
47.	Kanchan Lakhwani	133
48.	Kavitha Bhutada	135
49.	Keerthika	137
50.	Kiran Yadav	139
51.	Lalit Sharma	141
52.	Leena Lalwani	144
53.	Lipiie Banerjjee	146
54.	Madhu Soni	149
55.	Manissha Shah	152
56.	Mayur Ghate	155
57.	Mehul Gupta	157

58. Mini Baijal 159
59. Neelam Khemani 161
60. Neena Puri Nagpal 164
61. Neetu A Beel 167
62. Neha Piyush Nashine 169
63. Nidhi Chugh 172
64. Nimishaa Mathur 175
65. Nitender Mann 177
66. Om Prakash Priyadarshi 180
67. Pooja Gulati 183
68. Pooja Saxena 185
69. Pragya Sharma 188
70. Priyaa Chauhan 190
71. Priyanka Sapraa 193
72. Prof. Sarojini Gupta Biddanda 195
73. Promila Devi Sutharsan Huidrom 197
74. Punam Vishwkarma 199
75. Radhika Devgan 201
76. Raghunandan Chowdarapu 204
77. Rahul Churi 207
78. Reva Sarangal 209
79. Rita Sehgal 212
80. Rohan Jain 214
81. Rohet B Kummbar 217
82. Romi Maakan 220
83. Sadhana Athinamilagi 223
84. Sapna Gaurav Gupta 225
85. Sharlet Seraphim 226
86. Sheetal Pratik 229
87. Shelaj Kant 232
88. Shelly Arora 234
89. Shetall G Desai 236
90. Shikha Meher 239

91.	Shipra Goswami	241
92.	Shweta Singh	243
93.	Sri Rajeshwari Devi	245
94.	Sudha Krishnan	247
95.	Suvigya Seraphim Raj	249
96.	Suyog Patil	251
97.	Tanvee Kakati	254
98.	Tejjal Bhanshalii	257
99.	Trina Kanungo	260
100.	Uman Hooda	263
101.	Vaishali S Iyer	266
102.	Veena Chugh	268
103.	Veenu Mehendiratta	270
104.	Vijay Jain	272
105.	Vijayshri Panchikal	275
106.	Viji S	277
107.	Vinieta	279
108.	Vishal Sachdev	282
Blurb		285
Kindly Connect with Us		287
List of Books		288

Foreword by Nivedita Basu

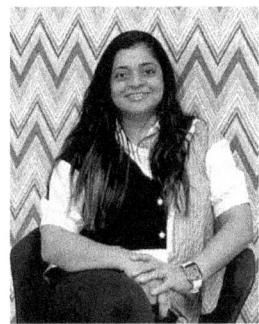
Life is a fascinating journey – a constant dance between what we learn, how we grow and what we expect from ourselves and the world around us. The very essence of this journey, with all its twists and turns, can often feel elusive. When I was invited to write the foreword for ***Seven LEE of Life,*** I was immediately captivated by the concept of distilling the wisdom of 108 visionaries into seven profound insights each, focused on ***Learning, Earning and Expectation.*** This is not just a book; it is a roadmap to navigating life's complexities with clarity and purpose.

What makes this anthology truly special is the sheer diversity of voices it contains. The 108 co-authors are individuals, who have lived, struggled, succeeded and, most importantly, learned. They come from all walks of life, bringing a wealth of experiences and perspectives that make this book a rich tapestry of wisdom. Every contributor has taken the time to encapsulate their life's lessons into seven meaningful takeaways – a task that is both daunting and courageous. They have shared not just their triumphs, but also their setbacks, each offering a unique lens through which to view the intricate dance of life.

The **"Seven LEE"** concept, which delves into ***Learning, Earning and Expectation,*** is both powerful and relevant. In a world that constantly demands more from us, it's easy to lose sight of what truly matters. Learning is the cornerstone of growth; Earning, beyond financial gain, speaks to the value we bring to the world; and Expectation, both from ourselves and others, shapes our reality. This book invites us to explore how these elements interact in our own lives, to reflect on our own journeys, and to gain clarity on what we want to achieve.

I believe that this book will not only inspire you but also encourage you to engage in introspection, to ask questions you may not have dared to ask before and to seek answers that are authentic to you. ***Seven LEE of Life*** is a celebration of the human spirit, of the drive to learn, to earn, and to set expectations that align with our deepest values. It is a reminder that we are not alone on this journey—our struggles, our dreams, and our hopes are echoed in the lives of others.

Congratulations to **Mrs Rainu Mangtani** and **Mr. Abhishaik Chitraans** and all involved in creating this anthology. May it inspire, challenge and guide you towards a more meaningful existence. Here's to the journey of learning, earning and expectation – we are all navigating together. I extend my deepest gratitude to the 108 contributors, who have courageously shared their wisdom.

With best wishes and blessings,

Nivedita Basu

Writer, Creative Director, Producer

Nivedita Basu is a well-known figure in the Indian Television Industry. She is living a happy married life with her caring husband Mr. Yadunath Bhargavan (Advocate) and also a lovely mother of a cute baby girl Oyshee Yadunath Karimbil. She has made a significant mark as a Producer, Creative Director and Content Developer. Over the years, she has worked on several popular TV shows and projects, playing a key role in shaping content for Indian television audiences.

Currently, as the Vice President of content, business alliances at **Atrangii Group** and owns a celebrity cricket team namely **Kolkata Baabu Moshayes** on the television reality show Box Cricket League.

Nivedita Basu is responsible for overseeing the creative direction, content development and programming strategies for the channel. Her background in the entertainment industry and experience with successful TV productions makes her a notable figure in the industry.

Foreword by Sidhharrth S Kumaar

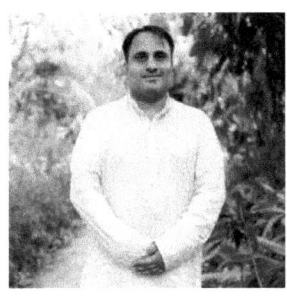
There are many learning, striving and hoping times in life. We change continually along the road, pursue our objectives and adjust our expectations. But suppose there was a way to reduce the core of this trip into seven fundamental ideas that would serve as our compass? Presenting the perspectives of 108 outstanding co-authors, each providing their individual insight on the pillars of **Learning, Earning** and **Expectation**, this massive anthology *Seven LEE of Life* provides exactly that.

This book is unique in that each author offers seven vital insights that build a strong framework covering the most important elements of our personal and professional life. Whether it's the lessons we discover in the demands of life, the quest of financial independence, or the expectations we create for others and ourselves, this anthology provides a thorough manual to grasp and control these essential components.

The variety of this book is its strength. With 108 voices, each from many walks of life, backgrounds and experiences, *Seven LEE of Life* offers a mosaic of viewpoints that is both rich and quite human. It asks us to examine our own path, ask ourselves how we measure success and think about how our expectations help to define our reality. It presents an ocean of ideas that lets the reader discover their own truth, their own road rather than a one-size-fits-all fix.

These pages will inspire, motivate and maybe even provide fresh perspective on the world. Each author's seven points are not only intellectual reflections but often result from actual experience hence they are all the more relevant and potent. Whether you're at the start of your road or far down the way, this book is a friend, a mentor, and a guide providing timeless knowledge much applicable to the difficulties of the modern society.

Seven LEE of Life is a transforming instrument rather than being an anthology of articles. It asks you to interact with its thoughts, consider your own experiences, and maybe come away with a new viewpoint on how to lead a meaningful and happy life. This anthology provides the tools to negotiate life with grace, resilience and purpose—regardless of your goals—learning more, making more money, or just establishing reasonable expectations.

As you explore the knowledge of these 108 geniuses, let their words motivate your own path. Discover your own road to a life well-lived by first picking what speaks to you, then challenging what doesn't.

With Love Light and Blessings,

Sidhharrth S Kumaar
Founder, NumroVani

Sidhharrth S Kumaar is a biopharma strategy consultant transformed into Astro Numerologist, Life & Relationship Coach, Energy Healer, Music Therapist and Brand Growth Consultant with a proven experience of around a decade.

He is the Founder & Chief Happiness Officer at **NumroVani,** who is on a mission to improve the happiness quotient in life by leveraging his proprietary 3P formula i.e. Proactive, Preventive and Personalized based on synergistic combination of Astrology, Numerology and Vedas with Modern Science.

He is known for innovations in baby name, wedding astrology and astrology for business. He has published 20+ research papers, 2 Books, and 20+ Research Guest Lectures at UGC- approved universities and has guided numerous people and brand in their growth journey. He also has one published patent in his credit and has guided people from all walks of life to become their best version.

Sidhharrth is also a TEDx Speaker (Youngest Numerologist globally to be one), Josh Talks Speaker, Fit India Champion and an avid writer on the subject. He has been felicitated with many recognitions, including the Times 40 U 40, ET Wedding Leader Award, Times of India Leaders of Tomorrow Award and Ayushcon Excellence Award.

॥ ॐ ॥

Foreword by Sneha

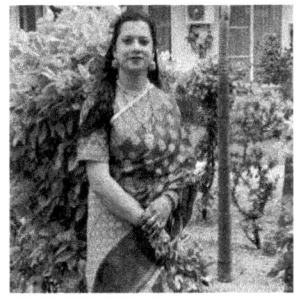

In *Seven LEE of Life,* this journey is exquisitely sketched out through a rare mix of knowledge and insight from 108 different voices, often compared to a road. But this book celebrates the complexity of life rather than only provides a set of life lessons. Offering readers something really special, it dares to probe big questions regarding our growth, prosperity, and future shaping.

Seven LEE of Life is brilliant mostly in its simplicity. Three fundamental elements of human life – **Learning, Earning** and **Expectation** – form the center of the book. Still, within this simplicity a world of complexity arises. Every one of the 108 writers organizes their great life events into seven main points of above three headings. Whether it's about overcoming obstacles, reaching achievement or reframing personal goals, these principles serve as stepping stones, directing the reader toward a fuller knowledge of life's several facets.

In an information-rich environment, what we most yearn for is clarity – and this anthology provides precisely that. These pages do not hide a one-size-fits-all formula or a big theory. Rather, it offers bite-sized pearls of knowledge that appeal at many phases of life. Whether you're just starting your career or looking back over decades of experience, there is something here that will really speak to you.

The most striking feature of this book is maybe its variety of voices. *Seven LEE of Life* ask readers to assume many diverse roles with authors from many walks of life, careers and cultural origins. This mosaic of viewpoints lets us grasp the common issues that mold everyone of us more broadly and richly. Every participant presents their own **'Seven Keys'** to life, therefore producing a symphony of ideas that appeal especially to each reader.

One does not approach reading *Seven LEE of Life* passively. It challenges you, invites you to reflect and interact. Though it has no simple solutions, it gives a range of insights that will enable you to probe your objectives, values and approach to both success and failure more effectively.

Fundamentally, this book is a personal development toolbox. Though it doesn't profess to have all the answers, it presents a broad spectrum of viewpoints that might guide your path. This anthology promises to be a consistent source of inspiration whether your search is for drive, clarity, or just a new perspective that you can go back to repeatedly.

Thus, use these pages slowly. Learn from the lessons, consider the tales and use the wisdom of these 108 visionaries to guide you. By doing this, you may simply discover your own **'Seven Keys'** to a successful, fulfilling life.

With the best wishes

Sneha

Founder, GrowthBeats Communications

Sneha is a management professional with around half a decade experience into People Management transformed into a relationship coach with proven experience of around half a decade in the same. She is Founder of **GrowthBeats Communication**s and Managing Chairman of **Haneeka Foundation**, where she devotes her time to women empowerment by facilitating health and education for girls and women all across globe. Sneha is also a mother of cute baby girl **Haneeka S Sandilya.**

॥ ॐ ॥

The Family of Visionary Co-authors

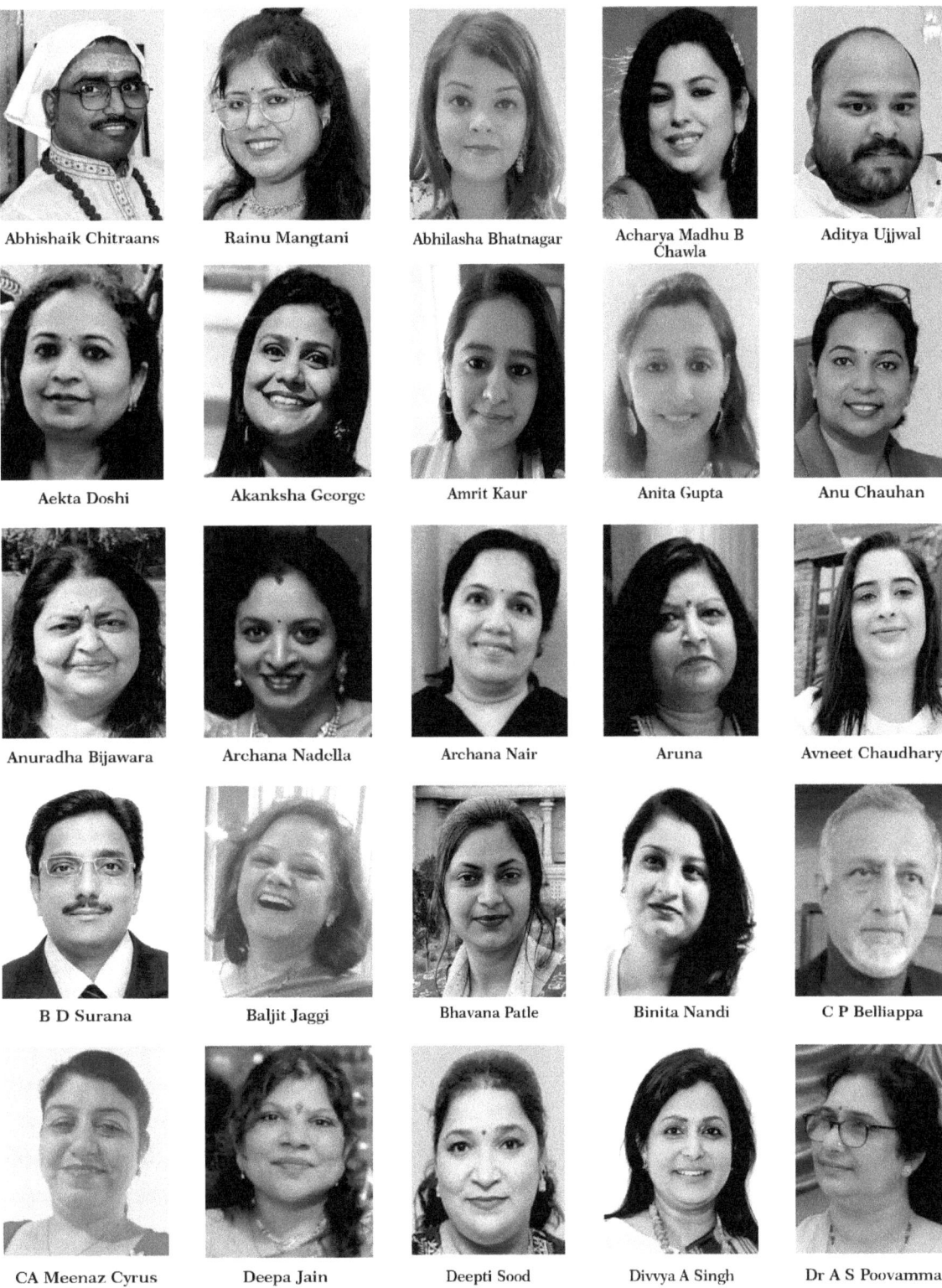

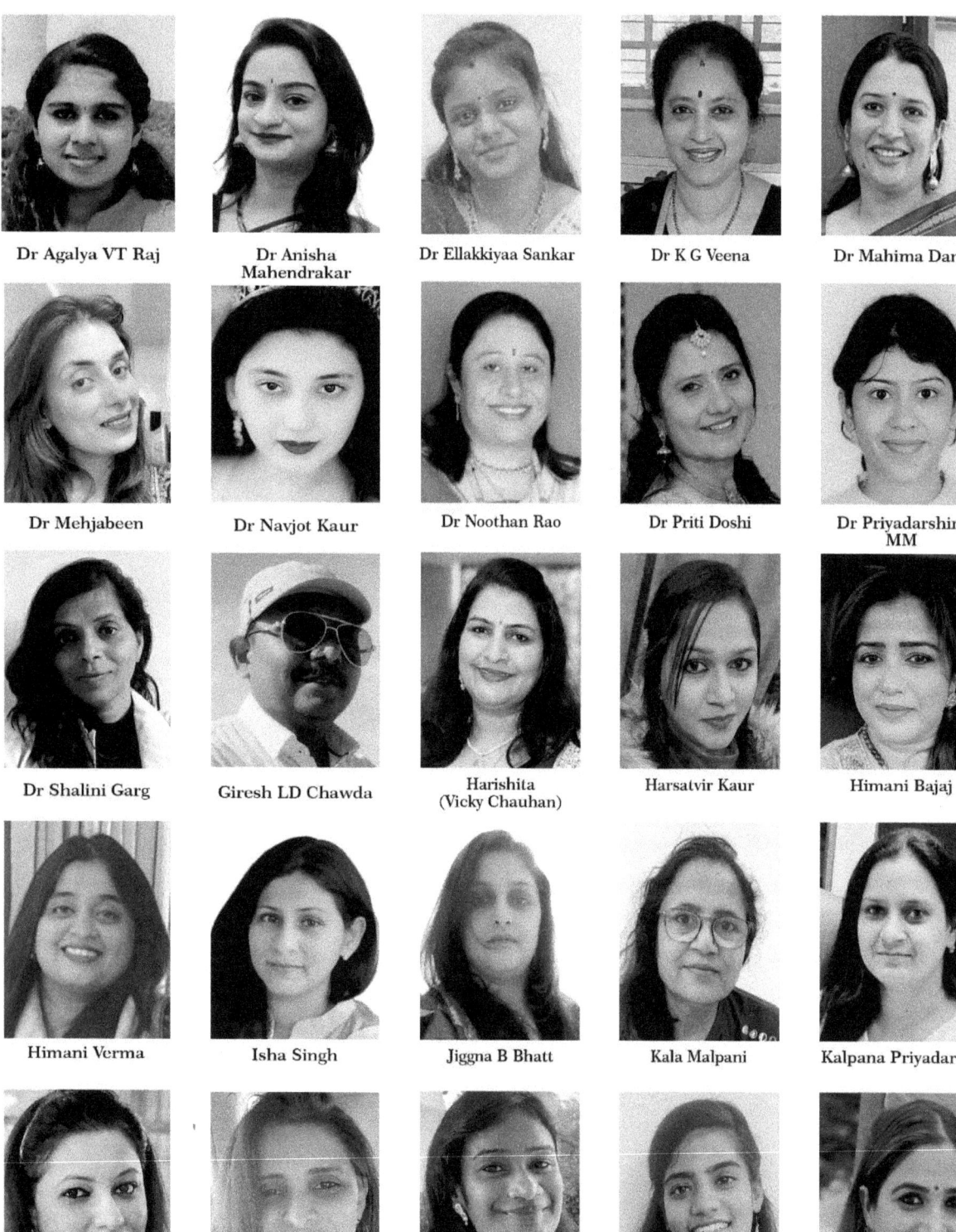

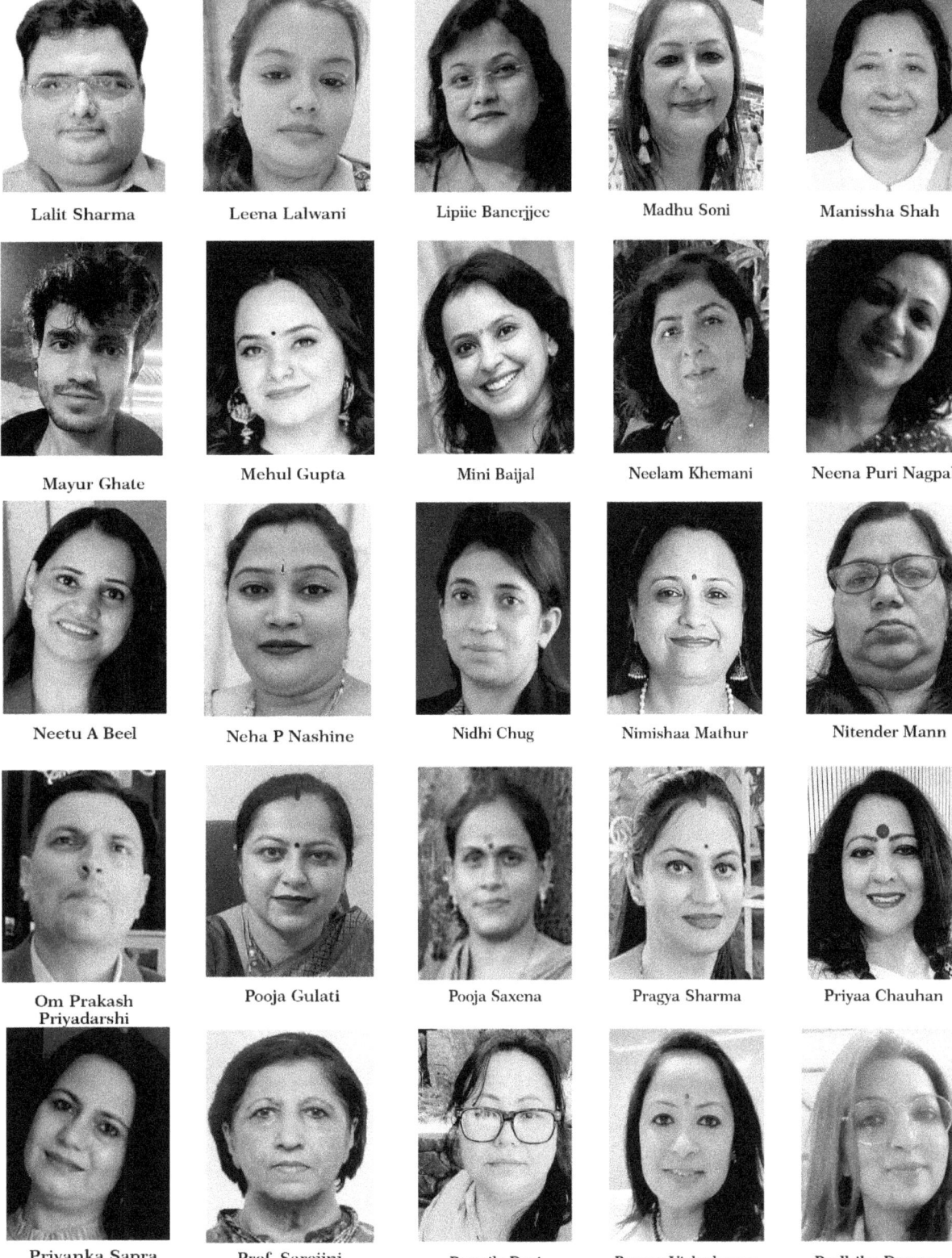

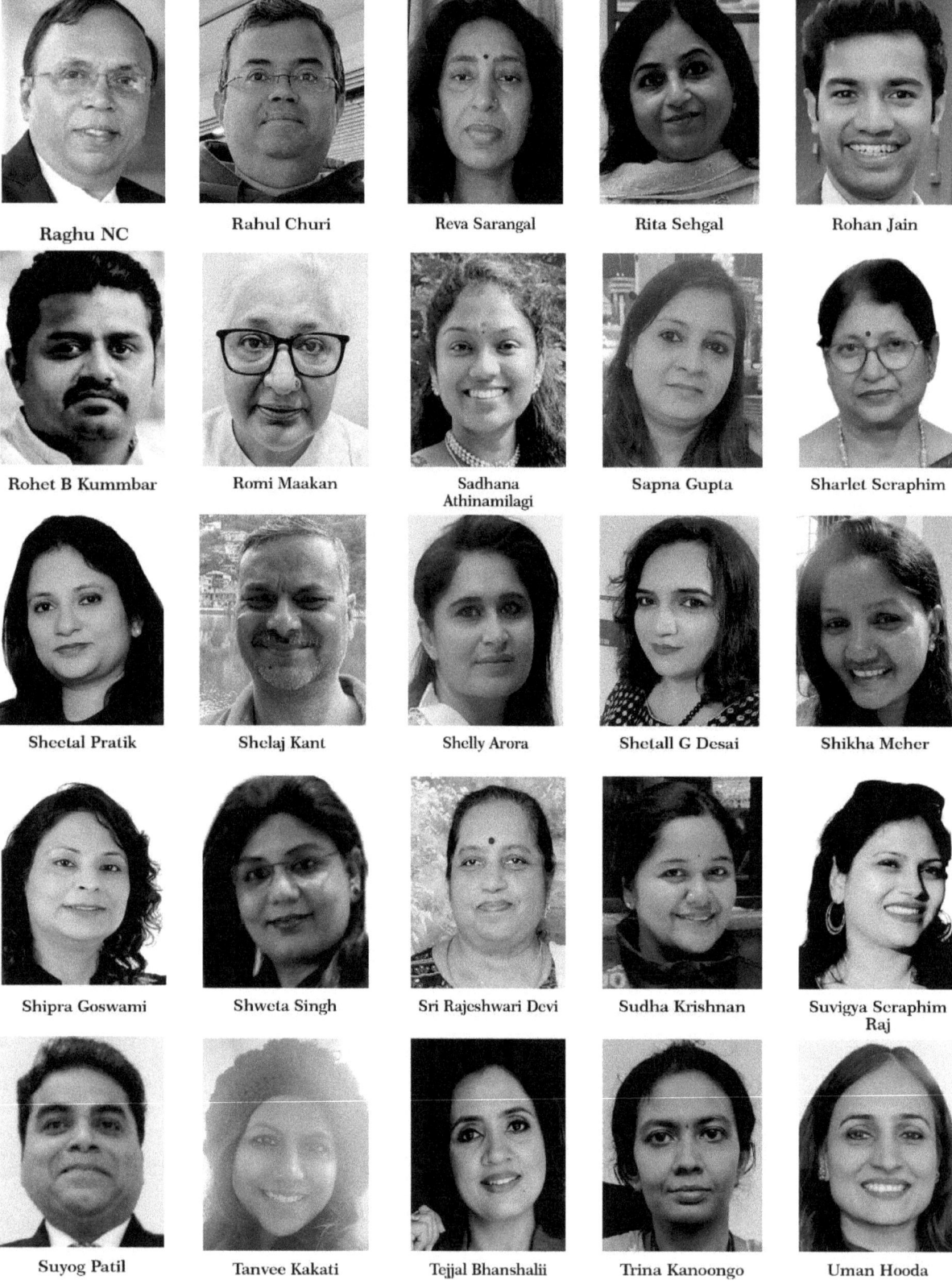

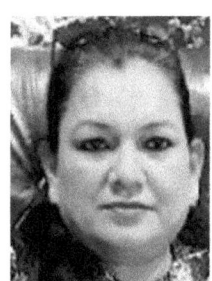 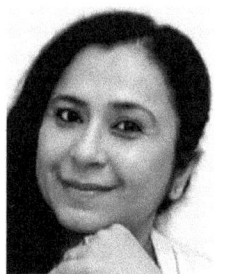 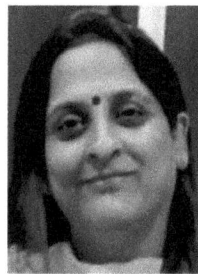 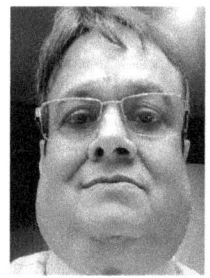 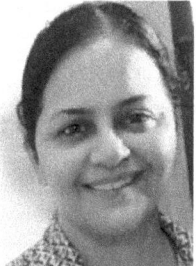

Vaishali S Iyer   Veena Chugh   Veenu Mehendiratta   Vijay Jain   Vijayshri Panchikal

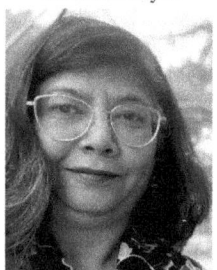 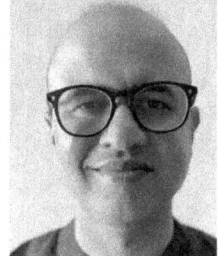

Vinieta   Vishal Sachdev

|| ॐ ||

Abhishaik Chitraans

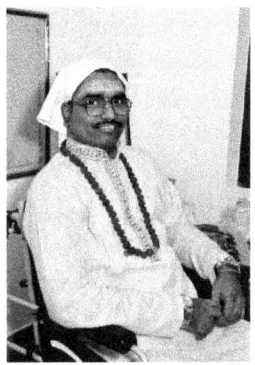

Abhishaik Chitraans is a distinguished numerologist, educator and internationally renowned published author, poet, expert columnist, philosopher as well as the visionary Founder and CEO of **Ankakshr Miracless,** *The Institute of Occult Sciences, Spiritual Activities and Research,* an institution registered by the Ministry of MSME, Government of India and Certified with ISO 9001:1015. Recognized by IVAF (International Vedic Astrology Federation) & AAA (Astrological Academic Alliances), USA. *Ankakshr Miracless* stands as a testament to Abhishaik's commitment to advancing numerology on a global scale. He is celebrated as the only numerologist worldwide to develop over five unique numerological formulas, combining the principles of BODMAS (mathematics) and physics to calculate life paths through date of birth. His contributions have set a new standard in numerology and his research has been published in over 10 international journals and prominent astrological magazines, including presentations at UGC-approved universities.

With three master's degrees in Commerce (M.Com.), Economics (M.A.) and Business Administration (MBA), Abhishaik brings a profound understanding of both academia and practical expertise. His professional journey spans more than a decade in high-level finance roles, including as Deputy General Manager of Accounts, Banking & Finance and an Internal Auditor with a top-10-ranked shipping cargo company in Africa and the Gulf region. However, his career took a remarkable turn in 2009, when he was diagnosed with *'Transverse Myelitis'***,** an untreatable condition that has left his lower limbs paralyzed. Despite this, he continues to excel and inspire, earning the moniker **'The Bed Traveller'** for his resilience and dedication to his life's mission.

In addition to his professional achievements, Abhishaik has become a Certified Professional Teacher, with a significant educational impact. He has guided over 1,000 Students/ Clients across 10+ countries, offering insights and consultations in numerology that span the globe. His published works include more than 30 articles on numerology and name numerology across leading magazines and online platforms.

Abhishaik's excellence and dedication have been widely recognized with numerous awards:

- World Record Holder for an International Poetry Anthology on Zodiac Signs
- First Prize in a state-level article writing competition by PCRA in Uttar Pradesh

- Excellence in Numerology & Research by ISA
- Jyotish Gaurav, Astro Diamond, Manavta Ratn, Vishisht Hindi Sewi, Sahitya Alankar Samman, Thai Sri Buddha Maharshi Award and Maharshi Agasthya Award etc.

Abhishaik Chitraans exemplifies resilience, knowledge and global influence in numerology, continually enriching the field with ground-breaking insights, innovative methodologies and a passion for transforming lives.

॥ ॐ ॥

Rainu Mangtani

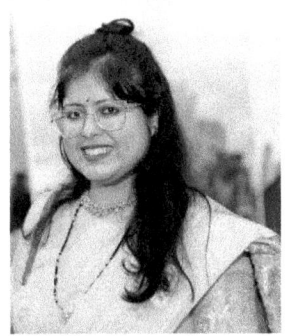

Rainu Mangtani, fondly known as *'The Versatile Iconic Personality'*, is a distinguished figure whose accomplishments span diverse fields, including banking, literature, content creation, and motivational speaking. A certified numerologist and graphologist with M.Com and IIBF Certification as a Digital Banker, Rainu has over six years of experience in the banking and insurance sectors, specializing in digital products for international clients and NRIs. Her professional expertise is matched by her impressive literary journey as a self-published and internationally recognized author, co-authoring over 25 books and compiling six anthologies that have highlighted over 500 voices.

Renowned for her dynamic presence, Rainu has graced multiple magazine covers, establishing herself as a true icon. She has been awarded titles such as *'Youth Icon'* by the Governor of Maharashtra and Asia's Top 30 Leading Women. She is an Expert Columnist, Best Author of the year 2022, Model Icon, Social Activist, World Record Holder, Perfect Author of year 2022, Best Content Writer of year 2023, Vlogger, The Celebrity Queen 2023, Brand Ambassador, Crown Girl, Speaker: Swell cast (Voice Over Artist). She's also the recipient of the prestigious National & International Dr APJ Abdul Kalam Awardee and got participation certificate for contributing her story to the world of cinema. As a finalist for CT Miss India International 2022, adding another dimension to her impressive repertoire recognized as *'The Celebrity Queen'*, a model and an inspirational figure.

Her works, *The Height of Life in 24 Rains, Today's Corporate World (A Robotic Mechanism of Youth)* and *Ladder of Success,* reflect her commitment to inspiring others

Rainu Mangtani is also a celebrated podcaster on **Ankakshr Miracless'** YouTube channel, a vlogger and an influential voice in the content creation realm. She uses this platform for empowerment and change, making her a beloved figure and an enduring *'Crown Girl'* in the public eyes.

|| ॐ ||

Seven LEE of Life
The Pillars

Compilers' Pen :

In *Seven LEE of Life,* we invite readers to journey through the insights of 108 visionaries, each offering a profound perspective on three pillars: *Learning, Earning* and *Expectation.* These elements our "**LEE**", are more than mere words; they represent a compass guiding us through personal growth, purpose and aspiration.

Learning is where it all begins. It's the continual process that shapes who we are and enables us to meet life's challenges with resilience. Through learning, we evolve, expand our minds and discover the endless possibilities life has to offer.

Earning goes beyond financial gain; it is the manifestation of our efforts, character and values. True earning reflects the legacy we build, allowing us to contribute meaningfully to the world around us and to find fulfillment in giving as much as we receive.

Expectation is the vision that keeps us moving forward. It challenges us to set higher goals, to believe in our potential and to reach for aspirations that push us beyond our limitations. Expectation is the bridge between our dreams and reality.

Together, *Learning, Earning* and *Expectation* form the foundation of a life lived with purpose and intention. Through the diverse voices in this book, we hope readers find inspiration, practical wisdom and a deeper understanding of the profound importance of these guiding principles in our journey of life.

> *"Learning inspires growth, earning rewards effort and expectation ignites the will to reach new heights."*

— **Rainu Mangtani**

— **Abhishaik Chitraans**

|| ॐ ||

Abhishaik Chitraans, a spirited soul from Bareilly (U.P) and **Rainu Mangtani**, a vivacious Mumbaikar are a match made in the Universe, tied together in love and companionship since June 2023. Their story began as two distinct worlds-colliding — Abhishaik's calm, introspective nature perfectly balancing Rainu's zest for life. Their lives have intertwined beautifully, combining the serenity of Abhishaik's spiritual mind-set with Rainu's vibrant personality. Since that fateful day they wed, they've woven a life that brims with love, laughter and a shared dedication to their work and beliefs. Their love is so profound that no argument ever holds them apart for long; when one is upset, the other finds a way to bring back joy, a testament to their unbreakable bond.

In February 2024, they made their mark at **World Book Fair**, Pragati Maidan, New Delhi, unveiling their much-acclaimed book, ***Deep Secrets of Name***, which explores advanced name numerology. The book captivated readers, offering insights into how names shape destinies, reflecting their dedication to spirituality and the occult sciences. United by their faith in God Shiva and Goddess Parwati, Abhishaik and Rainu embrace life's highs and lows with deep devotion and grace, bringing this spirit to their work at **Ankakshr Miracless**, *The Institute of Occult Sciences, Spiritual Activities and Research*, where, they guide others toward inner peace, balance, self-discovery, enlightenment and help individuals globally align with the universe's rhythm.

The newly married couple came up with the series of Anthology, where their first book with **51 co-authors** titled as '*Women Empowerment & Economic Developments*' was another hit and many more are on the way… As devout followers of God Shiva, Abhishaik and Rainu channel their faith into the work.

The couple also manages a popular YouTube channel namely **'Ankakshr Miracless'**, sharing knowledge and insights into numerology, spirituality and occult sciences, inspiring many to explore their inner selves through podcasts, reviews/ feedbacks and recording of online meetings and classes as well. Their passion for nurturing young talent led them to establish the '***Write-To-Earn***' community, where writers/ poets/ composers are rewarded for their contributions, fostering a space for creativity with a nominal annual registration as membership.

What is the actual reality behind their Love-Story and Life's Challenges?

Stay tuned to read soon…

॥ ॐ ॥

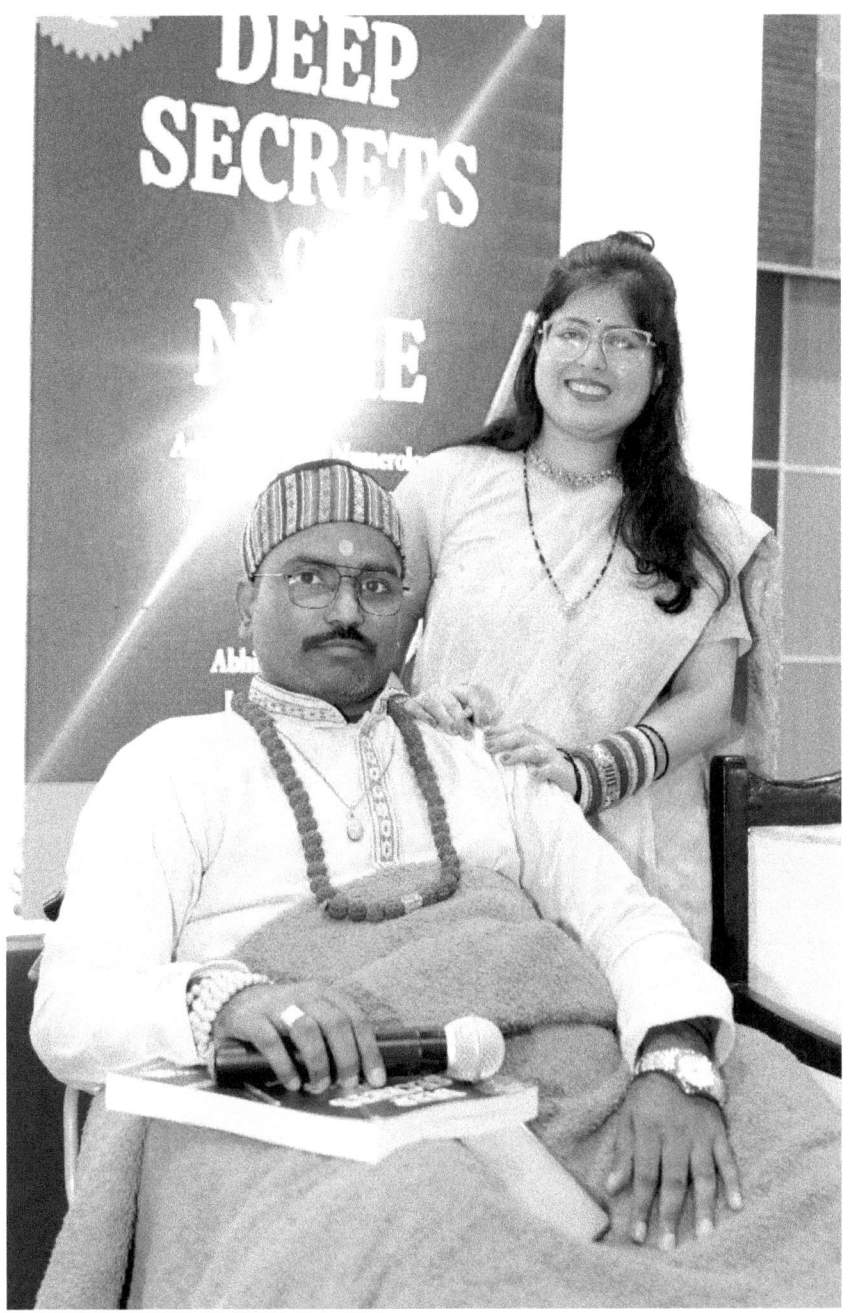

"Learning is the foundation, earning is the reward and expectation is the spark that attracts us toward our greatest achievements."

In *Seven LEE of Life*, renowned author couple cum compilers, Abhishaik Chitraans and Rainu Mangtani explore three foundational elements of life i.e. *Learning*, *Earning* and *Expectation* – that shape our life journeys.

Learning serves as the cornerstone, an on-going process that fosters adaptability, wisdom and growth. Through learning, we gain the skills and perspectives that guide us through life's complexities.

Earning represents holistic earnings as Love, Respect, Trust and Blessings.

Expectation is the subtle, driving force – both a motivator and a potential challenge. It urges us to strive higher, yet demands balance to avoid disappointment. Together, these three pillars create a rhythm, while this anthology reflects how aligning these principles can lead to a fulfilling, balanced life that honours both ambition and contentment.

Learning :

1. **Self-Discovery:** Life is an ongoing journey of self-exploration, helping one recognize strengths, weaknesses and unique potential.
2. **Acceptance and Letting Go**: Accepting life as it is and learning to let go of what cannot be changed is essential for peace.
3. **Learn from Failures:** Every failure is an opportunity for growth. Failures are Stepping Stones to Success.
4. **Rejection:** Behind every rejection there is some hidden golden opportunity and that's the universe's decision.
5. **Imperfections:** No one is Perfect in life !!!

    Not even you…. Yes, … You & We also… !!!
6. **Financial Struggles:** Times of financial hardship teach us resourcefulness, budgeting and the value of security.
7. **Comparison:** Never compare yourself to anyone, Stay real, Stay you… Keep it Simple, Try not to complicate.

These learning provide a blueprint for a balanced and fulfilled life, encouraging us to grow, connect and live with intention.

Earning:

1. **Trust:** It takes years and years to build it and just a second to break it.
2. **Respect:** Give Respect and Take Respect. It's a real earning which is beyond the words.
3. **Honesty:** Being Honest in life will automatically develop the trust and respect.
4. **Blessings:** Blessings of Universe and Elders are Magical and can turn your life into Heaven.
5. **Spirituality:** The Unconditional feeling of connecting with the supreme divine power.
6. **Patience:** Enduring with grace leads to wisdom and calm.
7. **Gratitude:** Thank you, thank you, thank you universe, for the beautiful human birth as it is in our fate after 84,00,000 species…

These principles enrich life, nurturing fulfilment, inner peace and strong relationships.

Expectation :

1. **Film Adaptations:** We want our exclusive story/ stories to turn into Film Adaptations and earn lots of love from the fans.

2. **Best Selling Author:** We are internationally renowned authors and soon we will be the Best-Selling authors worldwide.

3. **Financial Freedom & Prosperity:** We want to earn such a bulk amount to live our life with good worth and prosperity.

4. **World Travel:** We want to explore around the Globe.

5. **World Records:** We want to achieve the world records in our occult field then to the platforms that we are providing to our co-authors and much more.

6. **Happy, Healthy & Peaceful Life:** We are living a happy, healthy and peaceful life with our family and we want to continue to live the same as it is rightly said that **"Health is Wealth"**

7. **Iconic Influencer & Social Activist:** We want to become the popular influencers and social activists too.

Each expectation supports a holistic and fulfilling journey in life!

By integrating *Learning*, *Earning* and *Expectation* into our daily lives, we equip ourselves with the tools necessary for personal and professional growth. Embracing these pillars fosters resilience, drives success and leads us toward a life of fulfilment and purpose.

॥ ॐ ॥

Abhilasha Bhatnagar

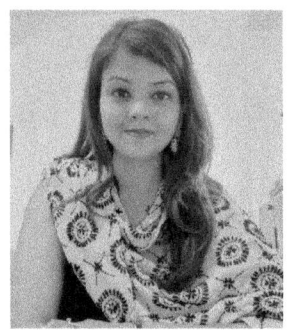

Author's Name	:	Abhilasha Bhatnagar
Qualification	:	M.Sc (Mathematics), M.Tech (IT), MCA, B.Sc Mathematics (Hons), B.Ed, CTET Qualified
Current Profession	:	Mathematics Facilitator
Age	:	38 years
E-mail ID	:	**bhatnagarabhilasha.17@gmail.com**
City/ Country	:	**Gurugram, India**

Abhilasha Bhatnagar is known for her strong academic achievements and creative talents, which highlight her dynamic personality and dedication to making a positive impact in education and culture. With triple Masters degrees in Mathematics (M.Sc.), Information Technology (M.Tech IT) and Computer Applications (MCA), along with a B.Ed. and CTET qualification, she exemplifies a deep commitment to education and continuous learning.

Her professional journey includes notable roles such as Lecturer at a college affiliated to IP University, Delhi and currently a Mathematics Facilitator, where she brings her expertise to inspire and educate students. Abhilasha is not only a proficient educator but also a budding author. She is also a recipient of the Global Teacher Award in 2021 by AKS Education Awards.

Her expertise extends beyond traditional teaching methods; she has been acclaimed as the "Online Teaching Supremo 2021" by Harper Collins, highlighting her innovative approach to digital education.

Outside academia, she is a multifaceted personality, having been crowned "Mrs. Congeniality 2015". She is also a travel enthusiast, who loves exploring new places and cultures.

Life is a beautiful gift from the supreme power. It is all about harmonizing **Learnings** for continually enhancing our knowledge and personality, **Earnings** not just for sustenance, but for satisfaction and managing **Expectations** to find balance and fulfillment. Each phase presents unique opportunities and challenges, shaping our personal and professional growth in numerous ways. Embracing lifelong learning helps us stay adaptable and resilient. Through this process, we discover the significance of relationships, the importance of perseverance, and the impact of empathy. We learn the most by life's experiences.

Learning:

1) One should have **Gratitude** of what you have, rather than focusing on what you do not have.

2) **Self-Love** should be practiced each day because the one who loves himself/herself can love other living beings as self-love enhances mental and physical health.

3) One should be **God-Fearing** because it instills moral responsibility, encourages good deeds, and promotes justice and fairness for all living beings.

4) There should always be a **Purpose** of life whether personal, professional, spiritual, or any other aspect

5) One should live with **Empathy** towards other living beings

6) One should always learn to **Give Back to the Society** by contributing positively to the community through various forms of support, service, or charitable actions.

7) One should learn the policy of **Forgive and Forget,** by letting go of anger towards someone who has wronged you and moving forward without holding onto negative emotions or grudges.

Earning:

1) **Self-Discovery** is most valuable earning in life that enriches personal growth, enhances self-awareness, clarifies values, and empowers individuals.

2) **Respect** is something which we earn in our life by doing good deeds and when we share our knowledge with others without expecting anything in return

3) **Love** of our near and dear ones

4) **Trust** of our family and our friends

5) Earn **Good Karmas** in life by doing good deeds to make future births peaceful

6) **Financial Stability** is a very important earning to ensure security, peace of mind, and the ability to pursue personal and professional goals. And to lead a comfortable and satisfactory life.

7) **Good Health** is a priceless earning that impacts every aspect of our life, ensuring we can live fully, achieve our dreams, and enjoy our journey to the fullest.

Expectation:

1) **Peace:** Everyone expects a peaceful life for themselves and their loved ones.

2) **Comfort:** People expect to find comfort in their personal and professional lives.

3) **Inner Satisfaction** is another thing which most of us expect should be there in our lives.

4) **Good Luck** is something which everyone desires in their lives

5) **Loving Family** is everyone's expectation and everyone deserves to have a loving and caring family.

6) **Supportive Friends** is another expectation of everyone from their lives. But of course, friendship is a two-way relation, so we all must be supportive if we expect support from our friends.

7) **Food, Clothes and Shelter** are the things which we all expect that we must have in our life for a comfortable and safe living.

|| ॐ ||

Acharya Madhu B Chawla

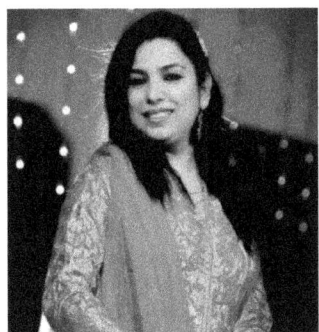

Author's Name	:	Acharya Madhu B Chawla
Qualification	:	M.B.A, MA in Astrology. Pursuing PHD
Current Profession	:	Numerologist & Astrology Consultant
Age	:	40 years
E-mail ID	:	**madhuchawlajpr@gmail.com**
City/ Country	:	**Jaipur, India**

Acharya Madhu B Chawla is a Renowned Astro-Numerologist from Jaipur Rajasthan, India, who specializes in using numerology to help individuals achieve their personal and professional goals. She has done her MBA. After that she has done Diploma from TISS-Mumbai on Child Protection & Diploma in CSR from Ministry of Corporate affairs. She had worked for 10 Years with NGOs & closely work & raise funds for many organizations & she was a trainer also. In 2016 she founded "Jeevan Sparsh Ngo" as she is keen interest & rich experience in development sector. She is into occult sciences since 2002, when she did Grand Master in Reiki in 2002. She has done Acharya (MA Astrology) and now Pursuing Phd In Astrology. She has great knowledge in different modalities like Numerology, Astrology, Vastu, Reiki.

She has mentored hundreds of students worldwide. She offers personalized consultations and coaching sessions to clients all over the world.

Acharya Madhu B Chawla believes that numbers are powerful tools for self-discovery and personal growth and she is dedicated to helping her clients unlock their full potential using the principles of numerology.

Madhu has the below LEEs of life :

Learning :

1) **Positive attitude** - I always think on the positive side rather negative

2) **Self Love** - If you can love yourself then others will automatically love you

3) **Choose your Words** - Language should have respect irrespective of any circumstances

4) **Never give up** - Whatever the situation is, never ever give up in life

5) **Do it Now** - Whatever we want to do we should do it now, tomorrow never comes

6) **Happiness** - To be happy within should be our own responsibility rather than expecting others to make us happy

7) **Responsibility** - Whatever is happening with us we should take the responsibility of that

Earning :

1) **People** - It's been said your network is your net worth, my people are my real assets

2) **Knowledge** - Since childhood I believe in gaining knowledge, this earning will be with me forever

3) **Love** - Love from my People is my real Earning

4) **Health** - Good Health is the real wealth in life

5) **Gratitude** - Gratitude always makes an abundance in my life

6) **Experience** - Experience of different things and travel makes me rich in knowledge and living a better life, and keeps me alive

7) **Wealth & Prosperity** - I believe in creating wealth so that if in my late days I am not earning I can live happily

Expectation:

1) **Be a Better Version of Myself** - I believe in Improving daily 1% to be a Better person

2) **Dreams** - To Have dreams and fulfill them

3) **Self-Motivation** - Motivation Is which always come from within, not outside

4) **Success** - I have to Be successful whatever task I choose for myself

5) **Love and Relationship** - In life there should be love, family, children and happy family

6) **Good Health** - I expect Good Physical and Mental health

7) **Financial Stability** - I expect financial Freedom and financial Stability

|| ॐ ||

Aditya Ujjwal

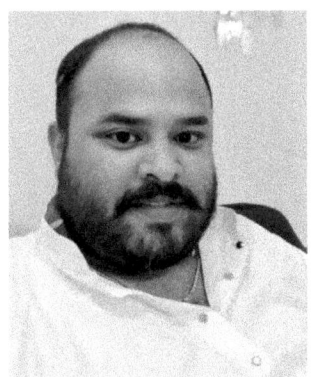

Author's Name	:	Aditya Ujjwal
Qualification	:	BBM, Masters in Astrology and Vastu
Current Profession	:	Businessman, Consultant
Age	:	31 years
E-mail ID	:	**adityaujwal7@gmail.com**
City/ Country	:	**Bangalore, India**

Aditya, hailing from Chapra, Bihar, holds a Bachelor's in Business Management (BBM) and a Master's Degree in Astrology and Vastu, showcasing his deep-rooted interest in spiritual sciences. Currently, he is expanding his knowledge by studying Numerology and Graphology. In addition to his academic pursuits,

Aditya is also a successful entrepreneur, running his e-commerce business, M/s Aditya Enterprises, which exports products internationally. His diverse expertise and entrepreneurial spirit make him a unique voice in the fields of spirituality and business.

Aditya has the below LEEs of life :

Learning :

1) **Positive attitude** - I always think on the positive side rather negative
2) **Self Love** - If you can love yourself then others will automatically love you
3) **Choose your Words**- Language should have respect irrespective of any circumstances
4) **Never give up** - Whatever the situation is, never ever give up in life

5) **Do it Now** - Whatever we want to do we should do it now, tomorrow never comes
6) **Happiness** - To be happy within should be our own responsibility rather than expecting others to make us happy
7) **Responsibility** - Whatever is happening with us we should take the responsibility of that

Earning :

1) **People** - It's been said your network is your net worth, my people are my real assets
2) **Knowledge** - Since childhood I believe in gaining knowledge, this earning will be with me forever
3) **Love** - Love from my People is my real Earning
4) **Health** - Good Health is the real wealth in life
5) **Gratitude** - Gratitude always makes an abundance in my life
6) **Experience** - Experience of different things and travel makes me rich in knowledge and living a better life, and keeps me alive
7) **Wealth & Prosperity** - I believe in creating wealth so that if in my late days I am not earning I can live happily

Expectation:

1) **Be a Better Version of Myself** - I believe in Improving daily 1% to be a Better person
2) **Dreams** - To Have dreams and fulfill them
3) **Self-Motivation** - Motivation Is which always come from within, not outside
4) **Success** - I have to Be successful whatever task I choose for myself
5) **Love and Relationship** - In life there should be love, family, children and happy family
6) **Good Health** - I expect Good Physical and Mental health
7) **Financial Stability** - I expect financial Freedom and financial Stability

|| ॐ ||

Aekta Doshi

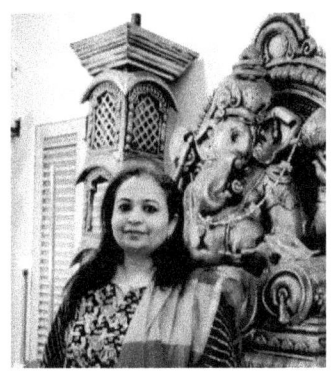

Author's Name	:	Aekta Doshi
Qualification	:	Home Science
Current Profession	:	Consultant and Counselor
Age	:	47 years
E-mail ID	:	**aad700@gmail.com**
City/ Country	:	**Mumbai, India**

Aekta Doshi has studied in Home Science followed by Diploma in Fashion Designing. She had been working in a Leading Garment Export house as a Merchandiser, but her family life & her passion for teaching made her an Entrepreneur and had established her Preschool Nursery for 6 years but due to health challenges it discontinued. After a break of 2 years she re-established her freelance academy namely "Edify Education" which trains Teachers through her experiences and prepare them to apply or establish their own academy. She also works as a Consultant in setting up Preschool Nursery & activity centre. She is a Graphologist, Handwriting expert and has authored cursive writing books for a publishing house and mentored to conduct Handwriting Competitions. Her passion for learning has driven her in the field of Occult Science. She is a Certified Numerologist, Bach Flower therapist, Tarot Card Reader, crystals and a remedial Vastu consultant and many more modalities as such for the betterment of the society.

Understanding of **'Seven LEE'** ie Learning, Earnings and Expectations are interconnected aspects of personal and professional growth, according to me is when you have a clear goal to achieve something there are many things around you which keeps on happening and you start observing the same. Seven is the most consolidated number there are many more to understand but if you make it principles of your life it can help you live better. When we are clear with some objective there is vast knowledge available around us through our good or bad experiences and if we try to find learnings from it is of great value. Life is journey and there are many expectations we have from it but each person has different experiences all together and unique learnings; when we fall in any wrong situations we need to focus on what is life trying to teach me; that helps you to grow into a matured person who can be an influencer to others. Any generation needs a good role model.

Learning :

1) **Self care & evolve in your thought process** – I strongly believe "Health is Wealth" and nothing is more important at the cost of your health.

2) **Fitness is root to happiness** – Ambitions and goals can be achieved and celebrated if you are fit.

3) **Embrace Failure and move on** – Embracing failure allows you to learn from your mistakes, grow stronger and develop resilience. Moving on from failure with a positive attitude is crucial for future success

4) **Value Relationships** - Meaningful relationships are necessary for our emotional support, happiness, and a sense of belonging.

5) **Practice Gratitude** - Gratitude shifts our focus and fosters positivity.

6) **Life long learning & self improvement**- Curiosity for seeking knowledge and self-improvement helps to stay engaged, adapt to change, and achieve personal and professional growth.

7) **Never compromise in your ethics** - Maintaining self-respect builds trust and ensures that our actions align with our values.

Earning :

1) **Career milestone** – achieved significant professional goals which provides a sense of accomplishment and financial independency.

2) **Wisdom, Knowledge and skills** - Wisdom comes from experience, while knowledge and skills can be acquired through education, it enables you to make good decisions.

3) **Patience and adaptability** - Developing the ability to remain patient and adapt to changing circumstances, helps to navigate challenges without losing our cool.

4) **Blessings** - A beautiful positive energy that flows in the form of blessings due to our actions and interactions.

5) **Take actions & responsibility** - Ideas and plans are essential, but execution matters most whether its pursuing a hobby maintaining relationship or practicing self care our actions shapes our future.

6) **Nurture relationship and network** – Nurturing our relationships and networks which are build on trust, empathy and mutually by investing time and efforts will cultivate and provide support whenever required.

7) **Various achievements which can add value to others life** - Success is just not defined as personal financial growth but its about contributing a positive impact in others life and leaving a lasting legacy.

Expectation :

1) **Respect and recognition -** Respect involves treating and valuing their opinions. Expecting to be valued for your contributions, efforts, and achievements, whether in personal, professional, or social contexts; appreciation gives a sense of worth from people around you. .

2) **Security & stability** - Feeling secure—emotionally, financially and physically is everyones desires.This encompasses having a reliable income, a safe living environment, and emotional security within relationships.

3) **Personal growth and development** - Evolving as a person through experiences and reflections expecting grow whether in skills, knowledge or character keeps us motivated.

4) **Meaningful Relationship** - Quality over quantity! Meaningful connections with family, friends and partners enrich our lives. These relationships offer emotional support, shared experiences and a sense of belonging.

5) **Balance & Harmony -** Harmony within our selves and with work, personal life, and health is crucial and our surroundings lead to contentment. This involves managing time and energy effectively to avoid burnout and maintain overall well-being.

6) **Purpose and contribution** - A sense of purpose through your passion or career gives life meaning and to contribute it positively to the world

7) **Spiritual fulfillment -** Spiritual fulfillment nourishes our soul. Seeking a deeper connection of unity, meaning & purpose with a higher power or finding inner peace and meaning through spiritual practices and exploring more to understand yourself and world around you.

|| ॐ ||

Akanksha Rebecca George

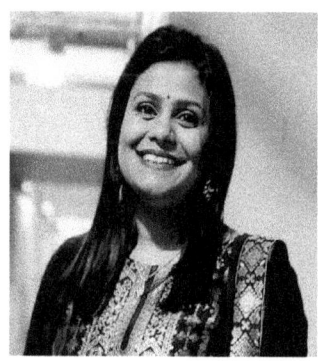

Author's Name	:	Akanksha Rebecca George
Qualification	:	B.Com., M.B.A.
Current Profession	:	Teacher, Avocational Writer
Age	:	36 years
E-mail ID	:	...
City/ Country	:	**Ghaziabad, India**

Akanksha Rebecca George is a wife and a mother of a boy. She is an orator and avocational writer. She has done her Bachelor of Commerce from Delhi University and completed her Master in Business Administration in Finance from SRM University.

After working a couple of months in the finance department of a prestigious organization, she realized her passion of imparting knowledge to others and her oratory skills. She started working as a corporate and soft skill trainer and then moved on to guide the children as per the education system. She is still working on molding the minds of children for a bright and fruitful life.

Life is a journey with problems to solve and lessons to learn but most of all experiences to enjoy and adventures to explore. Once a wise man was asked "What's the meaning of Life?" He replied, "Life itself has no meaning. Life is an opportunity to create meaning.". Life is from B (birth) to D (death). What letter lies between B and D? It's "C" which means Choice. Life is matter of choices. The road you take and the pace with which you ride is your choice. Your life is the result of the choices you make, if you don't like your life, it's time to start making better choices. Remember it's your road and yours alone, others may walk with you but no one can walk it for you. So, make the most of it.

Learning :

1) Health is the most valuable asset for survival so always appreciate, nurture and protect it.
2) Time is the most precious resource as lost time cannot come back.
3) Knowledge has a beginning but no end so keep learning as life never stops teaching.
4) You get what you give so treat others the way you want to be treated.
5) The only happiness that is satisfying and long lasting is the 'Happiness from within oneself'.
6) Patience is key to success
7) Life is too short, so live life to the fullest without wasting it on anger, worries, grudges and regrets.

Earning :

1) Money is not everything but money is something which is a very important part of life.
2) Respect which you earn when you give it over a lifetime with your act of kindness, honour & dignity.
3) Confidence and self-worth - outcomes of continuous learning & challenging yourself intellectually leading to personal growth and fulfilment.
4) One of the most expensive thing earned is trust as it takes years to earn it and seconds to lose it.
5) Relationships which are meaningful connections with family, friends and loved ones who enrich our life.
6) Good health
7) Happiness & sorrows based on our choices in life

Expectation :

1) To live life freely
2) To die healthy
3) To laugh more and spread happiness around
4) To be financially stable to enjoy life
5) To travel and explore the world
6) To see my child succeed in life
7) To make a difference in as many lives as I can and however I can.

|| ॐ ||

Amrit Kaur

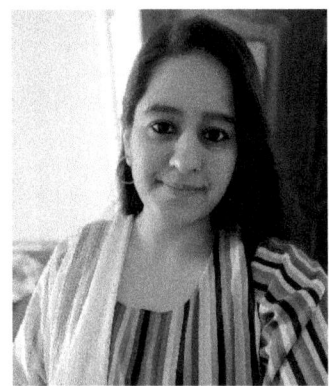

Author's Name	:	Amrit Kaur
Qualification	:	Diploma in Positive Mental Health
Current Profession	:	Tarot Card Reader & Vastu Consultant
Age	:	27 years
E-mail ID	:	**amritkaurmaan41@gmail.com**
City/ Country	:	**Pune Maharashtra, India**

VGM, Acharya Amrit Kaur, a 27-year-old author from Pune, Maharashtra, is a Professional Tarot Card Reader & Life Coach with over five years of experience. In 2024, she became the first youngest Vastu Grand Master & Vastu Acharya in Pune. She also won the **Indian Icon** of the Year award 2024 for becoming the best Vastu Consultant, Tarot Card Reader and Life Coach in Maharashtra.

I am 27 years old, and so far, what have I learned from myself? Despite the ups and downs in my life, I have remained steadfast in pursuing my goals. Before sharing my seven learnings, earnings, and expectations, I want to tell you that life is beautiful. Do not consider it tainted because of some sad moments. Because you have the ability to overcome challenges and achieve something new. It is true that facing every difficulty is not easy, but if we adopt certain principles in life, the journey becomes easier. I have learned that we desire 80% of the results out of 100% but only put in 20% of the work, we should not focus on the 80% result but on the 20% consistent effort. One day, this will surely give you 100% results. If I have achieved this, you will too. However, maintaining this requires determination; otherwise, despite your hard work, failure is inevitable.

Anyone can have the capacity to stand with us. However, it is essential to have the capacity to stand with yourself.

- **Amrit kaur**

Learning :

1) Don't hurry; be patient in every situation.
2) Ignore disrespect; just focus on your goals.
3) Don't seek revenge; just walk away.
4) Always stay motivated and confident in yourself.
5) Prioritize yourself with high standards.
6) Know your worth and value.
7) Take action for your rights.

Earning :

1) Find the purpose behind your thoughts and actions.
2) Take full control of your mental, physical, and emotional state.
3) Never judge yourself in any situation.
4) Don't be shy; ask for help when needed.
5) Don't beg; learn and earn for your life.
6) Avoid shortcuts; invest for the long term.
7) Don't be a servant if you are meant to be an emperor.

Expectation :

1) Freedom is your choice.
2) Improve knowledge and skills continually.
3) Be a multiplier of positivity and growth.
4) Have faith and show gratitude.
5) Listen to the universe and stay calm.
6) Don't lie or spy where not needed.
7) Make your own decisions.

|| ॐ ||

Anita Gupta

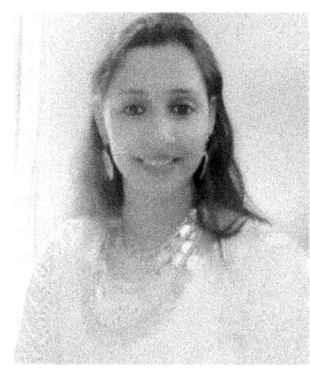

Author's Name	:	Anita Gupta
Qualification	:	M.A, B.Ed.
Current Profession	:	PYP Educator
Age	:	43 years
E-mail ID	:	**anitya1008@gmail.com**
City/ Country	:	**Gurgaon, India**

Anita Gupta, an IB PYP Educator at Delhi Public School, Ghaziabad Society, holds a Master's degree in Sociology from Banaras Hindu University along with a Bachelor of Education (B.Ed.) with extensive experience spanning over 15 years in teaching across various schools in Varanasi and Gurgaon. She is also trained in Nursery Education and proficient in educational technology. Anita is devoted to Lord Krishna and holds strong beliefs in spirituality.

'Life is a constant teacher, offering us new lessons every day. Our expectations shape these lessons, turning what we learn into valuable assets'.

As I've matured, I've come to hold fewer expectations from life. I've learned that true happiness stems from keeping these expectations modest. Expecting too much from others often leads to disappointment and hurt. Instead, I've found it more rewarding to set high expectations for myself. By striving to achieve my own aspirations, I've grown and learned that self-reliance and personal growth are the keys to fulfilment in life.

Learning :

1) **Faith in God**- Always trust in God because He always has a better plan for us.
2) **Prioritize family**- Never sacrifice your family's happiness to please outsiders.
3) **Embrace generosity**- Always share the knowledge you possess without hesitation.
4) **Express gratitude**- Always show gratitude to those who supported you during difficult times
5) **Strive through hard work**- The path of hard work may be challenging, but perseverance can reshape your destiny.
6) **Help the less fortunate**- Always contribute a portion of your earnings to those in need
7) **Count your blessings**- Karma is the ultimate reality, so conduct yourself in a manner that attracts blessings rather than curses.

Earning:

1) **God's blessings**- I've consistently felt God's blessings during challenging times.
2) **My family**- My family is my greatest strength; they have always stood by me, and their trust is my most valuable asset.
3) **My spouse**- Aditya is my greatest earning; I never imagined finding a life partner like him after experiencing difficult times.
4) **My Mentors & Friends**-I have been blessed with exceptional mentors and friens who consistently motivate and accept me for who I am.
5) **Students' affection**- As an educator, I am always surrounded by my students. While I earn money from my work, the love and affection I receive are more valuable than anything else.
6) **Contribute to the nation**-I am grateful to contribute to the next generation and serve the nation through my teaching.
7) **Source of income**- I am grateful to God for giving me the ability to earn money through my job and contribute towards fulfilling my dreams.

Expectation :

1) **Love**: I just want to spread love to everyone and hope for the same in return.
2) **Respect**: Respect women in relationships, families, and workplace
3) **Appreciation**: My productivity increases with motivation and appreciation. While monetary rewards are important, acknowledgment and recognition are equally effective motivators for me.
4) **Equality**: We women still face inequality compared to men, and this is what I expect society to address for all women.
5) **Peace**: To sustain national growth, I appeal for peace and expect peace from our country.

6) **Money**: Money is essential for a good life, although it's materialistic. As a teacher, I believe that salaries in this profession are inadequate. I expect better compensation for educators.

7) **Blessings**: If I do something good, I hope for blessings from that person rather than criticism behind my back.

॥ ॐ ॥

Anu Chauhan

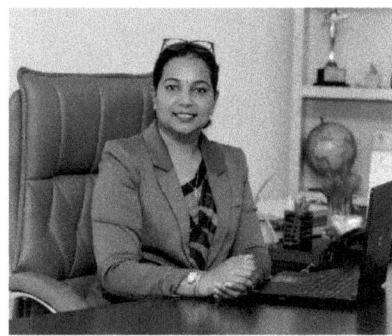

Author's Name	:	Anu Chauhan
Qualification	:	B.Com., M.B.A,
Current Profession	:	Educationist and Trainer
Age	:	41 years
E-mail ID	:	**anuchauhanfp@gmail.com**
City/ Country	:	**Gurugram, India**

Anu Chauhan is an educationist with a specialization in Eary Years with more than 14 years of experience. She is an entrepreneur and running a successful pre-school in the heart of Gurgaon since last 8 years. She holds a Master Degree in Business Management. She has worked with reputed Bank for years and moved to renowned educational institutes after realizing her passion towards learning & development of young learners. She has a passion to empower new parents.

She is a teacher and a trainer empowering Eary Years Educators with the access of new possibilities. She believes that learning is a never ending process and with that passion she is deeply invested in transforming teachers & child development in early years.

'Seven LEE of Life' will make you be present to yourself. You will introspect and retrospect your life helping yourself to have a better understanding of where you are and where you are heading to. You will begin to focus on your feelings and emotions and start analysing your past experiences. Resulting in self-growth and self-improvement, here I am sharing the Seven LEEs of my life

Learning :

1) **Be Grateful** – Being grateful is the source of true power. It is where you will find your true strength.

2) **Strength** – Difficulties in your life don't come to destroy you but to make you realize your full potential.

3) **Be Humble** – Humanity is underrated. Being humble is an important skill as it keeps you grounded, teachable regardless of how much you already have or know.

4) **Be Positive** – your thoughts have power & thinking is the greatest power we possess. Use it wisely.

5) **Character** – A good reputation is more valuable than money.

6) **Keep Trying** – You never loose until you stop trying. Choose "I'll try" over 'I can't".

7) **Be a Giver** – The more you give the more you receive. Success doesn't count from how much you get but from how much you give.

Earning :

1) **My Family** – my strength, my strong pillar of life with unconditional love and support.

2) **My Daughter** – the greatest earning of my life. She is the direct blessing of god telling me that I have to be a better person, a strong mother whom she can look up-to.

3) **My Mother** – she incepted the seed of compassion in me. I am in debt to her for raising me and teaching me to operate with love and compassion.

4) **My Flock** – I am blessed to have people in my life who love and respect me unconditionally.

5) **Spirituality** – I am grateful to be a little enlightened to be spiritually evoked by the blessings of my guru.

6) **My State of Being** – I am humble, respectful, grateful, accepted, loved and empowered.

7) **Being Alive** – Rather then in virtue of my existence, I am thankful for being alive.

Expectation :

1) **Be Fearless** – I will try to bounce back with my failed attempts. If I succeed good, if not I will not blame anyone.

2) **Explore** – Break my comfort zone and explore the possibilities.

3) **Dream Big** – Work hard to make them into reality.

4) **Time Management** – We all have 24 hours to us. Make best out of it.

5) **Be meaningful** – Have purpose in life.

6) **Resentment** – leave it behind and create your own heaven

7) **Creating Healthy Boundaries** – learn to create healthy boundaries for self care and emotional health.

|| ॐ ||

Anuradha Bijawara

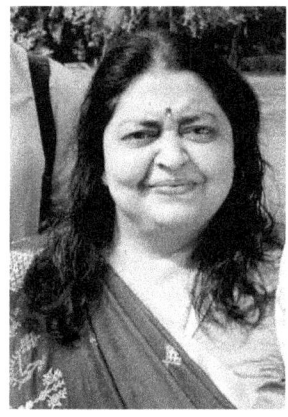

Author's Name	:	Anuradha Bijawara
Qualification	:	Graduate
Current Profession	:	Acupressure Therapist
Age	:	49 Years
E-mail ID	:	**anuradhasree09@gmail.com**
City/ Country	:	**Bangalore, India**

Anuradha Bijawara is a lovable home maker. Passionate story teller and an Acupressure Therapist. She is a B.A. graduate with lots of interest in social work. She has helped her nephew, who is hearing her impaired boy to learn speech and his studies.

After dedicating her 28 years of her family, now wants to pursue her passion. She is also animal lover, especially street dogs and has also adopted 6 dogs in her street and plans to start an NGO for street dogs along with her son, She is an excellent cook also.

Anuradha is a patient listener and extrovert, a reliable friend and is loved by everyone in her neighbourhood.

This topic **'Seven LEE of Life'** is essential fore-ground to anybody's Life **First L** stands for **Learning, E** stands for **Earning** and another **E stands for Expectation**. As humans, if we follow seven essence of life, then our birth will be – Worthwhile.

Anuradha's seven LEEs are as follows:

Learning :

1. **Confidence:** By learning one gets confidence On oneself
2. **Personal Development:** Learning brings inner development in you
3. **New Opportunities:** Through Learning new opportunities opens up in front of you eg: job, education & business.
4. **Problem Solving:** Learning makes you more intelligent as to face and Solve any problem in your life
5. **Knowledge is Power:** Learning is is the only power which can never be taken away, knowledge is for eternity
6. **Ready for the Unexpected:** Be ready to face any challenges in Life
7. **Improve your Mental Health:** Learning makes your mind more active than being Idle.

Earning :

1. **Social:** earnings which is ethical in behaviour.
2. **Material:** Monetary benefits you get from money
3. **Personal:** Your caring, sharing and respecting other human is personal earning
4. **Physical:** How well maintain your physical health is also earning
5. **Religious:** Being Spiritual is also earning
6. **Family:** Maintaining good relationship with all your family members is also your earning
7. **Knowledge:** Earning of Knowledge is the only earning which possess with us for life time.

Expectation :

1. **From Life:** Peace and Contentment
2. **From family:** Understanding and cooperation with one and all.
3. **From Society:** Good environment and equality
4. **From self:** Pure mind and Selflessness
5. **From Learning:** Gain knowledge and Overall development of mind and body
6. **From Earning:** Monetary benefits and satisfactory Living
7. **From Government:** Security, basic needs for day to day Living

According to me these above said are the ultimate examples of *Seven LEE of Life*.

|| ॐ ||

Archana Nadella

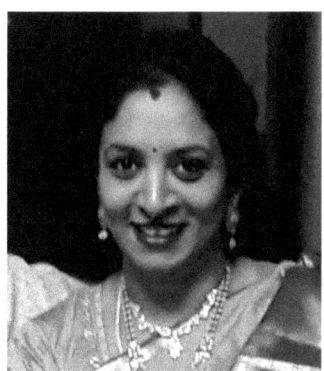

Author's Name	:	Archana Nadella
Qualification	:	B.Com., MBA (General Management)
Current Profession	:	Healer and Therapist
Age	:	49 years
E-mail ID	:	**na.archanaa@gmail.com**
City/ Country	:	**Bangalore, India**

Archana Nadella is an Internationally Certified Handwriting Analyst & a Graphotherapist. She has done her Graduation in Commerce and Post-Graduation in General Management. She has a worked as admin with few organizations and as a Senior Personal Loan Officer at a renowned MNC Bank.

Archana Nadella, has acquired several skills sets in various healing modalities and been certified as a counselor from few renowned counseling centers. She has closely worked as associates with several other practitioners to adept and strengthen her knowledge. Always have worked one on one personally as she believed in giving complete attention, however with the necessities being dissimilar is now slowly expanding and extending to make a big opening in the field.

Archana Nadella, has trained several individuals to have a tailored personality and healed and counselled several issues.

Learn Earn and Return this is what I have heard and have grown today the concept is Learning, Earning and Expecting. Initially, I got little perplexed thinking that learning and earning is still ok, but what is this expecting? I thought it is about expecting from others earnings from others, but a after little thought I understood it's about me, myself and Archana (ARCHIE).

I took pretty long time to go through all the learnings from my life and what I have earned out of it and what I am expecting out of it and I was amazed and thrilled to understand that outer journey is very simple compared to the inner journey. The opening that has happened in this process of introspection is profound and I think each and every one should try this process and see what's the result are revealing for themselves.

Learning :

1) **Enriching:** enriches every bit of a human cell is what I felt
2) **Experience:** life is experienced best when you learn every moment
3) **Encompassing:** every aspect teaches if you are open with all senses
4) **Empowering:** power is existing with all, but learning empowers.
5) **Evolving:** you evolve with every new learning
6) **Eloquent:** a human start becoming free flow like a river
7) **Empathetic:** we grow compassionate with every learning

Earning :

1) **Amused:** earning forever fun and bliss is what one earns
2) **Acclaimed:** you are accepted with so much of renown
3) **Acknowledged:** brecognition is free in air
4) **Admired:** super liked by all
5) **Amazed:** get treated with utmost astonishment
6) **Attuned:** connection with HIGH is simple
7) **Attained:** 24/7, 365 days you feel complete

Expectation :

1) **Stability:** attain almost stillness in everything
2) **Sustainability:** resource of almost anything and everything
3) **Support:** you not only become your own system, but extend to others too easily.
4) **Serenity:** calmness throughout
5) **Salient:** prominence is your exuberance
6) **Security:** sense of protection in all ways
7) **Sagely:** becoming nonjudgmental and getting wiser

|| ॐ ||

Archana Nair

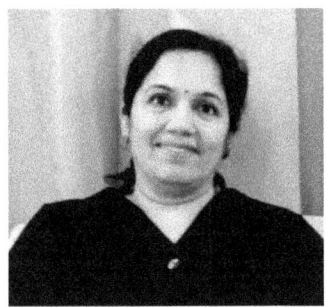

Author's Name	:	Archana Nair
Qualification	:	M.B.A., M.Sc. (Applied Psychology)
		PG Diploma in Counseling
Current Profession	:	Lecturer in Management, Corporate Trainer, Management Consultant, Counseling Psychologist
Age	:	50 years
E-mail ID	:	**archana.nairkr@gmail.com**
City/ Country	:	**Cochin, India**

Archana Nair has been teaching Management at the university level since, 1998. She serves as a project guide for management students in undergraduate, postgraduate and M.Phil courses. She is a member of the Board of Examinations at Universities in Kerala and has published several papers on Integrated Marketing Communication in both international and national journals.

The author also holds M.Sc. degree in Applied Psychology with a Post Graduate diploma in counselling, she has been involved in counseling for over 15 years. Archana is a hypnotherapist and a graphotherapist for the past three years.

As a trainer, she provides training to various corporate offices, teachers, students, and individuals from all walks of life. The author is the Managing Director of TU Consultors Pvt. Ltd, where she supervises market feasibility studies for many FMCG products as a Management Consultant. Archana Nair is one of the leading trainers in NLP and has successfully trained 20 batches of trainees.

The impact of learning is reflected in what a person earns through their acquired knowledge. This extends beyond material wealth, encompassing a holistic view of what makes life meaningful and fulfilling. The quality of one's friends and positive traits —such as attitude, adaptability and credibility – serve as true indicators of life's rewards.

Life's expectations can become obstacles between learning and earning if not properly managed. Unrealistic expectations can lead to disappointment when they don't align with one's capacity for growth. Ultimately, those who absorb the right lessons lay a strong foundation for their learning and achieve greater success in life.

Learning :

1. Love yourself to feel loved by others
2. Don't withhold your emotions, express them and you'll feel better.
3. Please don't forget to breathe when you're angry.
4. Be kind and stop judging others.
5. Treat people with respect so that people may repay you at a great price.
6. Always weigh your words before firing them out.
7. Be laid back and stress free.

Earning :

1. The quality and depth of relationships with family, friends and colleagues.
2. Emotional and mental well-being through the sense of happiness, contentment, and mental health that results from positive life choices and experiences.
3. The ability to balance professional and personal life, leading to overall happiness and fulfilment in various aspects of life.
4. The practice of being present in the moment, which can lead to deeper appreciation of life and its simple pleasures.
5. Developing adaptability to face challenges in life.
6. Understanding and appreciating diverse perspectives, cultures, and communities, leading to personal growth and empathy.
7. Spiritual fulfilment, leading to a deeper sense of purpose

Expectation :

1. Financial stability and growth to meet materialistic needs.
2. Career goals as the first result of acquiring knowledge.
3. The desire for fulfilling relationships, including friendships, romantic partnerships, and family connections
4. Pursuing personal dreams and aspirations, related to career, hobbies, or personal passions.
5. Contribute to the community and engage in socially responsible behaviour.

6. Anticipating good health and a long life, often leading to lifestyle choices aimed at wellness.
7. The belief that one should be happy and find meaning in life, which can create pressure to achieve certain emotional states.

｜｜ ॐ ｜｜

Aruna

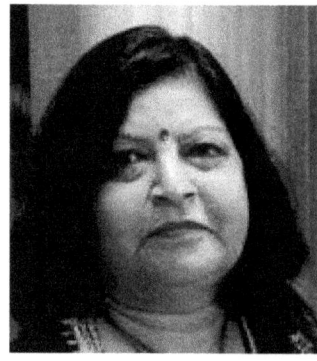

Author's Name	:	Aruna
Qualification	:	B.A., L.L.B
Current Profession	:	Artist and Freelancer
Age	:	64 years
E-mail ID	:	**arunachaudhary19@gmail.com**
City/ Country	:	**Gurugram, India**

Aruna is a multifaceted homemaker, blending her professional expertise as a lawyer with her artistic passion. As a freelancer, she constantly explores new business ideas, driven by her inquisitive nature. A well-traveled soul, she delights in experiencing diverse cultures and cuisines. An avid reader and natural teacher, Aruna's spiritual inclination draws her to the tranquility of nature. She finds immense joy in spreading happiness, using her rich life experiences to motivate and inspire others.

Aruna's unique combination of skills, creativity and positivity makes her a captivating and insightful author, offering a wealth of knowledge and inspiration.

In the intricate tapestry of life, certain guiding principles light our path towards personal growth, meaningful relationships, and enduring happiness. This article delves into the seven key areas of learning, earning, and expecting that shape my journey. These core values – patience, sincerity, goodness, self-love, clarity, forgiveness, and positive thinking – serve as foundational pillars for personal development and enriched experiences. Our adherence to these principles influences how we interact with others and how we find purpose and joy in our lives. As we navigate through learning and earning, these values guide us towards a fulfilling existence. By understanding and applying these essential principles, we create a framework for achieving a balanced life filled with meaningful connections and enduring contentment.

Learning :

1) **Patience: Patience allows everyone to accomplish tasks gracefully.**
2) **Sincerity:** One must be sincere to achieve their goals
3) **Goodness:** Acts of goodness never go waste; they always return in kind.
4) **Love:** Love yourself first, for only then can you truly love others.
5) **Clarity:** It is essential to have clear goals.
6) **Forgiveness:** Forgiveness lightens the heart and frees the soul
7) **Positive Thinking:** Positive thinking leads you down the right path in life.

Earning :

1) **Goodwill:** I have earned the goodwill of my friends.
2) **Friendship:** I have a few, but very sincere friends.
3) **Loyalty:** My loved ones are exceptionally loyal to me.
4) **Trust:** The trust of my friends and relatives is invaluable.
5) **Respect:** My good conduct consistently earns me respect in my circle.
6) **Gratitude:** My close ones always express their gratitude for my timely help.
7) **Faithfulness:** People are faithful to me because of my upright conduct.

Expectation :

1) **Peace:** I seek peace in all my relationships.
2) **Financial Stability:** I desire financial stability in my life.
3) **Good Friends:** I hope to always have good friends by my side.
4) **Decency:** I wish for people to behave with decency.
5) **Happiness:** I love to have happiness around me.
6) **Smiles:** I want to see beautiful smiles on people's faces.
7) **Reputation:** I strive to have a good reputation among those who know me.

|| ॐ ||

Avneet Chaudhary

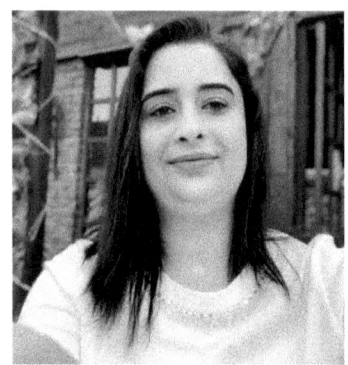

Author's Name	:	Avneet Chaudhary
Qualification	:	B.A., M.B.A. (HR & Marketing)
Current Profession	:	Teacher, Painter, Influencer, Entrepreneur, Homemaker
Age	:	36 years
E-mail ID	:	**avneet6choudhary@gmail.com**
City/ Country	:	**Gurugram, India**

Avneet Chaudhary is self-managed personality. She is a proficient entrepreneur ,painter. Avneet is a dedicated and resourceful homemaker with the passion for creating a warm and organised home environment .She believes that a well-managed home is the foundation of a happy and productive family life. Feels great joy nurturing her family and ensuring that home is welcoming space for everyone.

Openness friendliness thoughtfulness emotional stability are features of our personality singing cooking reading are her passion.

Avneet Chaudhary has the below LEEs of life :

Learning :

1. **Perspective** – Perspective is how we recognise the opportunities and make life best out of them.
2. **Flexibility** – Impact fulfilment in all areas of life flexibility in hurdles and create success in life.
3. **Patience** – Ability of tolerance in negative situations, which protects the behaviour from negative attitude.
4. **Uncertainty** – Unpredictable clashes between heart and mind with situation.

5. **Balance** – If you know what when and how approach to achieving a fulfilling and balanced life.
6. **Forgiveness** – Important to relax your anger towards someone's mistakes for self mental peace.
7. **Adjustment** – A balance between expectation and what actually happens in life.

Earning :

1. **Self-love** – loving yourself before loving others teach the best way to enjoy life .
2. **Family/ Responsibilities** – Family is sport comfort advice values culture also responsibilities, sacrifice for loved ones.
3. **Trust** – Trust is the belief that life has a way of unfolding can lead to growth learning and positive outcomes.
4. **Happiness** – Happiness depends on the quality of our thoughts deeply personal and multifaceted experiences.
5. **Personality** – A unique combination of behaviours and thoughts, interactions shaping one's character.
6. **Respect** – It is the greatest experience of love for self-personality by others.
7. **Experiences** – Life lessons we get in our whole journey gives a vision to see this world more reflectively.

Expectation :

1. **Health is the wealth** – Maintaining physical and mental health to boast energy at different levels.
2. **Peacefulness** – Your life must need to surround yourself with supportive and positive people.
3. **Freedom** – The ability to live according own values desires and choices while balancing the constraints of society.
4. **Money** – Of course very important to meet our needs, facilitate with economic strength.
5. **Stability** – Stability is the key component to professional and emotional success and well being
6. **Successful** – A combination of our achievements in personal and professional life impacts that on society.
7. **Opportunities** – Life demand is identifying and seizing favourable situation to achieve life gaol.

|| ॐ ||

B D Surana

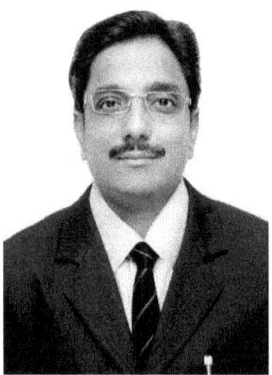

Author's Name	:	B D Surana
Qualification	:	B.Com (Hon) CA (Inter) Certified Graphologist and Counselor
Current Profession	:	HR & Management Consultant, Stock Sub Broker, Trainer, Graphologist, Social Worker
Age	:	58 years
E-mail ID	:	**bdsurana@gmail.com**
City/ Country	:	**Kolkata, India**

B D Surana is SEBI authorised AP. His Education is B.Com (Hons.), CA Finalist, Accounting Certificate from ICAI. Diploma in Counselling & Psychotherapy, MILT Leadership Course, Leadership in Recruitment, Mind Training etc., Advance Level Certification in Graphology, Scientific Logos, Face Reading, Watch Analysis etc.

He is attached with several Professional and Social Organisations like Lions International, holding various important positions and have received many awards and recognitions. He is a life member of JITO, ISTD, NIPM, NHRD, MILT, All India Marwari Sangh, RSFF, Chinmoy Mission and other bodies.

B D Surana is associated with HR Business as Founder & Chief Consultant at Surana Equity Pvt. Ltd. For more than 26 years. (www.hrequity.in)

Life is beautiful. Life is opportunity. Life is preparedness. We leave our impression. We built our personality & leave behind mark. We built aura and impress world. We must learn & make others learn to fight to save our generations, traditions, society, family & culture. We must observe world

& culture. Reading books is things required in life to learn from experience, research & hard work of writers, authors, poets etc. My personal experience is anyone who is in learning path , nobody can defeat that person , because knowledge is key to success & you can earn with the knowledge & ideas. Now I share my **Seven LEEs of Life** as under

Learning :

1) **Expectation:** No Expectation from others
2) **Listening:** Toughest thing in life
3) **Rich:** Rich mentality is more important than monetarily rich
4) **Focus:** Laser Focus is more important in life
5) **Thought:** Always be on learning mode than on old thought pattern
6) **Goal:** Without fixed goal you cant reach any where
7) **Build:** Build thing more than you consume

Earning:

1) **Self-Made** – My biggest earning is I am self-made
2) **Sincere** – What work I take up I take sincerely
3) **Discipline** – I try to maintain discipline , even when nobody looking
4) **Straight forward** – I am very straight forward in dealing with people
5) **Courage** – I am courageous and take appropriate risks
6) **Leader** – People say leaders are born but I have earned it
7) **Self-Learner** – I learn new things always

Expectation:

1) **Happy** – I want happy all time
2) **Peace** – I want peace of mind
3) **Rich** – Born Poor Die Rich
4) **Help** – Help in need is help in deed
5) **Give back** – I want to give back to society
6) **Growth** – I want to see India as growth country
7) **Challenges** – I love to give challenges

|| ॐ ||

Baljit Jaggi

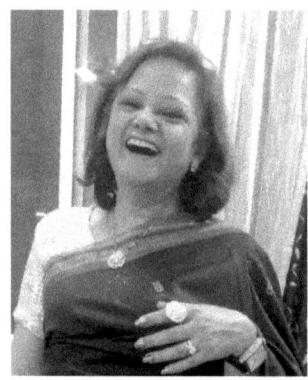

Author's Name	:	Baljit Jaggi
Qualification	:	B. Com, M.B.A,
Current Profession	:	Life Coach & Healer
Age	:	54 years
E-mail ID	:	**winningbells@gmail.com**
City/ Country	:	**Pune, India**

Baljit Jaggi is a budding Author, Certified Coach & a Ho'oponopono Healer, whose mission is to facilitate in transforming 100,000 lives. She has done her Master in Business Administration and Advanced Diploma in Marketing & Sales. She has worked for more than 5 years as Director for an Event Management company providing customized solutions to Top Notch Corporate Houses & also worked as Corporate Trainer for more than 7 years providing training, from Bharat Ratna Organizations like BPCL, NTPC, ONGC to MNCs like Nestle, Coco-Cola, Hindustan Levers Ltd., Honda Motors, HDFC-SLIC to Top National companies like Reliance Infocomm., Maruti Udyog Ltd, SBI, Indian Railways, VSGM and many other.

Also contributed as an Academic Counselor with a MNC for more than 3 years and began her career as a teacher. She has been an avid trekker and a sports lover, dabs her fingers in sketching & painting sometimes and loves cooking occasionally. She is a nature lover plus a kitabi Keera!! She is happily married to Col. K.S Jaggi of Indian Army.

Learning, Earning and Expectation are one of the main Aspects of Life for which we Live our Life and walk on the Progress Path of Life. Learning teaches us how to take our Journey of Life by Learning New Things each and every Day. Who is a Student? answer is Every Human Being is a Student as we learn something New Each and Every Day. Learning leads us to Earnings and

Expectations in our Life Journey. Proper Earning leads to proper Investments and our Earnings leads to proper Investments and Our Earnings and Investments Fulfils are Expectations in Life. When we Fulfil our Expectations in Life we feel Happy, Joyes, Satisfied and Successful in Life. TO conclude Learning, Earning and Expectations are related with each other.

Learning :

1) **Endless:** There is no end to your learning, new learning and relearning in your entire life.

2) **Every Day:** In Your Life Journey you learn something new every day.

3) **Guidance:** Learning should ne taken as Guidance for Life.

4) **Motivational:** Every Day Learing should be a motivation for Life Path.

5) **Correction:** Learning should be a corrective measure for our past mistakes.

6) **Mistake:** Whenever You make mistake in life take it as Learning Experience so that you do not repeat the same again.

7) **Abundance:** Learning should be used in a proper way to bring Abundance of Knowledge in Life.

Earning :

1) **Earning:** Earning should me minimum Four Times than your Spending.

2) **Spending:** Only Small Amount of Earning should be spend.

3) **Investments:** Investments of Majority Earnings should be done in such a way that in Long Term Returns are Multifold.

4) **Abundance:** Earnings should bring n Abundance flow of Income in Life.

5) **Multisource:** Earnings should be from Multiple sources so that the Expansion in Investments become Faster.

6) **Multifold:** Earngins should be Multifold to Increase the Wealth.

7) **Gratitude:** Earning should be welcomed in Life with Gratitude.

Expectation :

1) **Successful:** To be successful Spiritually and Mentally.

2) **Abundance:** Abundance Money wise, Health wise

3) **Family:** Family should be Loving, Caring and Understanding amongst each Member.

4) **Spouse:** Spouse should be such a person who is matured enough to handle each and every situation in Married Life.

5) **Maturity:** One should handle situations and challenges that arouse in Life in a Matured way day by day.

6) **Peacful:** Entire Life Journey should be a peaceful Journey. This is possible if one gives time for a low phase to pass through Life Cycle.

7) **Expectation:** Life Should be full of Abundance, Love Joy and Happiness.

॥ ॐ ॥

Bhavana M Patle

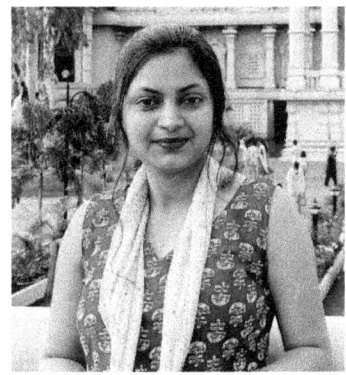

Author's Name	:	Bhavana M Patle
Qualification	:	B.B.A., M.B.A. (HR)
Current Profession	:	Data Analyst, Content Writer
Age	:	24 years
E-mail ID	:	**bhavi1111patle@gmail.com**
City/ Country	:	**Nagpur, Maharashtra, India**

Bhavana Patle is a Certified Data Analyst and Data scientist. She is a budding poet she wrote poems in Marathi and Hindi, English as well on love, spirituality, fun, self-love & care etc. she is writing articles on self-awareness, ancient taboos for women's or individual persons mental health & care. She is also interested in Psychology and Numerology, Yoga/Exercising, Reading.

Bhavana Patle is professionally working as Team Lead & Data Analyst in Government organization known as Mahatma Jyotiba Phule Training and Research Institution (MAHAJYOTI), Nagpur. She is Fun Loving, Spiritual and kind Person Also Started Travelling in Maharashtra, many more to Explore. She Participated in Career Counselling Programs with Colombia Maxim Institutions, Digital marketing programs.

Learn & Earn, for example if I am able to perform any process as data analyst it's because of learning and I am able to earn money just because of learning. Learning is reciprocal of Earning, in between if you expect something from anyone it will hurt you but you may expect from yourself (believe in yourself) it will develop a desiring mind set (इच्छुक मानसिकता) then you can do anything that is impossible.

Learning is acquiring knowledge, skills & understanding and continuous learning help you to grow personally, mentally, emotionally, spiritually. Earning is important for financial stability and sustaining a desired lifestyle. Expectation is beliefs or assumptions about what is going to happen in future in your life.

In my survey, I found some want to be successful in life by using knowledge or some are just cheating with themselves by using others; Personally, I felt everyone holding hidden talent the only thing is missing is clear learning of own self (knowing yourself) that's why people are failing in life.

'Before expecting from ourselves we need to know ourselves'

'Know yourself, learn & earn.'

'Learning is Power to earn and fill void vault with full of expectations from your growing self'

Learning:

1) Learning will make you shine.

2) It is Never Ending Web (जाल)

3) Learning new things hits new gain or opportunity.

4) Learning is weapon to earn money and respect in infinite way.

5) Suffering is learning.

6) Man becomes omniscient (सर्वज्ञ) by spreading knowledge

7) Learning is affluence (ख़ज़ाना) that will follow you till end of life

Earning:

1) Earning will make you fine.
2) If you are consistent for anything, it's your earning.
3) Earning lead to quality of life.
4) Save money like a camel saves water.
5) Absolutely Needful to live in Kalyug (कलयुग).
6) Earning is a valuable thing that makes people befriend you.
7) Earning respect along with the money is more important.

Expectation:

1) Expecting will make you align towards Goals.
2) Expectations lie between 2Es (education & earning).
3) Your personality is a shadow of your expectations.
4) Expecting money is equal to legacy in life
5) Don't rely on others to fulfill your expectations.

6) Be silent when you full of expectation and work on it.

7) Expectations is root of happiness & heartbreak as well.

"Learn, Earn and Achieve: Set Expectations, Exceed Goals"

॥ ॐ ॥

Binita Nandi

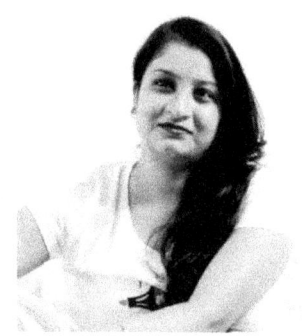

Author's Name	:	Binita Nandi
Qualification	:	M.Sc.
Current Profession	:	Career Strategist and Life Coach
Age	:	43 years
E-mail ID	:	**success.nitanandi@gmail.com**
City/ Country	:	**Hyderabad, India**

Binita Nandi is a Life Coach, Parenting Coach, Career strategist, DMIT (Dermatoglyphics Multiple Intelligence Test) analyst, certified Numerologist and NLP master practitioner. She has done her Master Degree in Science. She has started her career in 2008 as a Counselor in the Dept. of Health and Family Welfare in State Govt. of West Bengal. As a parenting coach, she has helped many parents on positive parenting to gain a better understanding of their parental journey.

Binita Nandi is the founder and CEO of Happy Life Society. It is the one stop solution for life's four major parameters as Health, Relationship, Career and Spirituality. Mission of Happy Life Society is to help people to become an emotionally content, economically fulfilling and physically healthy and their best version in terms of developing happy and thriving societies.

Our life is our best teacher. Everything we learn along the way in life becomes the actual learning for our future. Everyday, every moment of life is teaching us something or the other, that education is the container and career in our ongoing life.

We have certain expectations towards life. We keep ourselves busy in various ways to fulfil those expectations. We learn different things from every task and that is our actual earnings of life.

The wisdom gained from the teacher called Life is the ultimate gain in our life, and this earning shows us the right direction by saving us from various mistakes and we also able to understand life correctly.

Learning :

1. **Journey** – Life is a journey, not a destination.
2. **Value** – Time is our more valuable resource.
3. **Focus** – Always be focused in own task.
4. **Invest** – Invest time and support towards relationship.
5. **Accept** – Accept changes and truth easily.
6. **Love** – Happiness is love.
7. **Try** – Never fail to try more.

Earning :

1. **Health** – Health is wealth, so always take care.
2. **Enjoy** – Enjoy every moment of the life.
3. **Relationship** – Earn the relationship with empathy, sensitivity and kindness.
4. **Belief** – Belief that you are beautiful.
5. **Problem Solving** – Every problem has its own solution.
6. **Gratitude** – Appreciate everything that what I have now.
7. **Openness** – Be open to learning to new things.

Expectation :

1. **Opportunities** –Try to grab every opportunity and take action to make it successful.
2. **Help** – Help needy people, help society.
3. **Forgiveness** – Learn to forgive others and self also.
4. **Balance** – Balancing my need or desire for flexibility of life and set priorities accordingly.
5. **Freedom** – Having the freedom to find and pursue my "True Purpose" in life.
6. **Fulfilment** – Utilising my potential in the best possible way, for myself and for others.
7. **Stability** – Figuring out what to do next, to keep a float and be a bridge to my later years and retirement.

|| ॐ ||

C P Belliappa

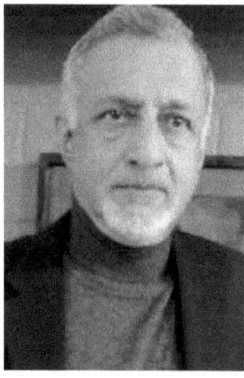

Author's Name	:	C. P. Belliappa
Qualification	:	M.E. (Chem. Eng)
Current Profession	:	Agriculture
Age	:	78 years
E-mail ID	:	**bellicp@yahoo.com**
City/ Country	:	**Karnataka, India**

C. P. Belliappa is a chemical engineer. After working for companies such as Indian Oil Corporation, Rallis India, and Humphreys & Glasgow Consultants, he returned to his hometown in Kodagu, in Karnataka where he manages his coffee plantation.

Belliappa is an educationist, a pragmatist, a rationalist, and a Darwinian evolutionist. Writing is his hobby. He has written numerous articles and essays in leading newspapers, magazines, and websites. Rupa Publications has published 5 books authored by Belliappa.

Life of modern humans can be encapsulated under three important categories viz., Learning, Earning and Expectation (LEE).

Each of these three categories can be divided into seven subcategories. Listed below are my points to elaborate on the LEE of human life. Those who plan and practice the Seven LEEs of Life effectively can expect success in education and success in their adult lives as earning members. Successful individuals not only contribute to their family's well-being but also add to the wealth of the nation. Everyone desires and expects a happy and fulfilling life. By following the Seven LEEs of life it is possible to achieve one's ambitions and goals in life.

Learning :

1. Learning is a lifelong journey that enriches our minds and broadens our horizons.
2. Learning gives us the knowledge and skills needed to navigate and succeed in an ever-changing world.
3. Curiosity lights the flame of learning.
4. Learning from our mistakes is a powerful way to grow and improve.
5. Sharing knowledge with others enhances the learning experience.
6. New challenges and ideas are essential for meaningful learning.
7. There is joy in learning and in discovering new concepts.

Earning :

1. Earning provides financial stability.
2. Diversifying income sources can enhance financial security.
3. Sound education and skills development can significantly improve earning potential.
4. Financial planning and judicious saving are crucial for long-term wealth accumulation.
5. Responsible entrepreneurship can provide much higher earnings though risks exist.
6. Steady income streams, such as fixed deposits, rental properties, and stock market, can supplement income.
7. Balancing work and family life is crucial in ensuring the pursuit of wealth does not compromise well-being.

Expectation :

1. Expectations improve our perceptions and influence our achievements.
2. Unrealistic expectations often lead to disappointment and frustration.
3. Managing expectations involves balancing optimism with realism.
4. Expectations can motivate individuals to achieve goals and strive for further improvement.
5. Adjusting expectations in changing circumstances is crucial for positive results.
6. Mutual respect and understanding are essential for meeting expectations in relationships.
7. Candid communication of expectations prevents misunderstandings and conflicts.

|| ॐ ||

CA Meenaz Cyrus Surty

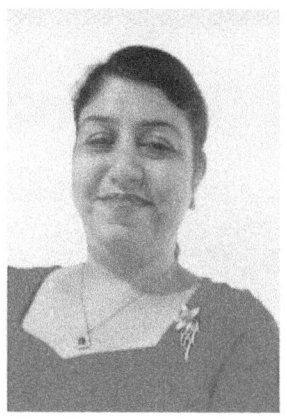

Author's Name	:	CA Meenaz Cyrus Surty
Qualification	:	B.Com., C.A.
Current Profession	:	Service in Government Sector Consultant and Counselor in Occult Science
Age	:	51 years
E-mail ID	:	**meenaz.surty@gmail.com**
City/ Country	:	**Surat, India**

Meenaz is a Chartered Accountant by profession. She was a ranker throughout her school days and had a bright academic career. She has completed her silver jubilee (25 years) in her profession with wide range of experience in private and government sector. At present she is serving as an officer in a semi government organisation.

In the field of occult science, she has acquired knowledge in Automatic Writing, Angel Card Reading, Access Consciousness Bars Practitioner, Numerology, Handwriting Analysis, Crystal, Healing through frequency and artificial intelligence and many more modalities like Spirit Animals, Dream Analysis, etc. She specialises in Talk Therapy and is eager to learn Mediumship. She considers herself as life-long learner. She is the founder of "MYSTICAL MEENAZ- Follow your Heart", a brand where she practises all her healing, spiritual and occult modalities.

Learning, Earning and expectation are interconnected aspects of personal growth and development. Learning fosters knowledge and skill acquisition, leading to increased earning potential and expanded career opportunities. As we learn, our expectations for ourselves and our lives naturally expand. However, it's essential to balance expectations with reality, avoiding unrealistic goals that can lead to disappointment and frustration. By setting achievable expectations, we can harness the power of learning and earning to drive progress and fulfilment. This balance enables us to learn, earn, and expect with clarity, leading to a more satisfying and purposeful life. Effective balance is the key to a happy and productive life.

The journey of learning unfolds with each new day. We earn knowledge and wisdom along the way. Eventually, expectations rise and goals come into sight. The roots of learning grow deep and lay a strong foundation of life. As skills are learned, our earning potential blooms. Together, they harmonise and give a purpose, growth and fulfilment to our life.

The seven points are from the initial letters of the words **Learning, Earning** and **Expectation;**

Learning :

L – Literacy : Literacy is the foundation of lifelong learning empowering individuals to access knowledge, communicate effectively and participate fully in their communities.

E – Education : Education is the key to unlocking individual potential, fostering personal growth and transforming lives, communities and societies for the better.

A – Academics : Academics lay the groundwork for future success, providing a foundation of knowledge and skills that propel individuals toward their goals.

R – Research : Research ignites curiosity, fuels discovery and expands knowledge, driving innovation and progress in various fields of study.

N – Note Taking : Effective note taking enhances learning, retention and recall, helping individuals process and retain information and study more efficiently.

I – Inquiry : Inquiry sparks curiosity, encouraging learners to explore, investigate and discover knowledge through active questioning and critical thinking.

G – Growth : Habits of lifelong learning foster continuous growth, empowering individuals to adapt, evolve, and reach their full potential.

Earning :

E – Entrepreneurship : Entrepreneurship fuels innovation, creativity and economic growth, empowering individuals to turn their passions into successful businesses and create value in the market.

A – Assets : Building and managing valuable assets such as investments or property, can generate passive income and create long-term financial security.

R – Revenue : Increasing revenue through strategic sales, marketing and customer growth is crucial for businesses to achieve profitability and sustain long-term success.

N – Net Worth : Building a strong net worth through smart financial decisions, investments and debt management provides a foundation for long-term financial stability and security.

I – Investments : Making informed and strategic investments can help grow wealth, diversify income streams and secure long-term financial goals such as retirement or legacy planning.

N – Negotiation : Effective negotiation skills can significantly impact the earning potential as they enable individuals to confidently advocate for fair compensation, benefits and opportunities that align with their value and worth.

G – Gains : Realising significant gains from investments or business ventures can lead to substantial financial growth and a notable increase in net worth.

Expectation :

X – X-Factor : The presence of an X-factor can significantly impact the outcome of a situation, often exceeding expectations and leading to surprising and unexpected results.

P – Possibility : Recognizing the possibility of multiple outcomes can help manage expectations, allowing for a more flexible and adaptable approach to achieving goals and handling unexpected results.

E – Envision : To effectively plan for the future, it's essential to envision what you want to achieve and set clear goals that align with your values and aspirations.

C – Confidence : Having confidence in your abilities and preparation can boost your expectations and lead to outstanding achievements, as a positive mindset can drive success and fuel accomplishment.

T – Target : Setting clear targets helps align expectations with achievable goals, providing a focused direction and increasing the likelihood of success.

A – Anticipation : Building anticipation can heighten expectations, creating a sense of excitement and eagerness for a future event or outcome and potentially leading to a more fulfilling experience.

I – Insight : Gaining insight into a situation can adjust and refine expectations, allowing for a more informed and realistic understanding of what to anticipate and how to prepare.

|| ॐ ||

Deepa Jain

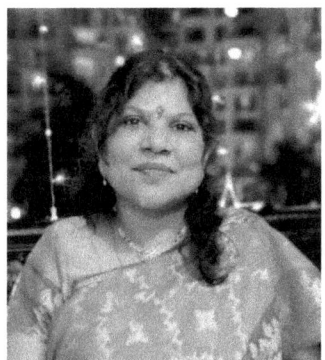

Author's Name	:	Deepa Jain
Qualification	:	B. Com., Course in Public Speaking
Current Profession	:	Home Maker, Helping Hand of Husband
Age	:	52 years
E-mail ID	:	**deepasuren1995@gmail.com**
City/ Country	:	**Mumbai, India**

Deepa Jain is skilled in house management and helping hand of her life partner, sharing his responsibilities as an entrepreneur in the field of banking and correspondence. She always had a keen interest in penning down her deep thoughts in form of poems and stories. She also takes interest in dance, music, meditation etc. She is good counsellor too.

Deepa Jain has the below LEEs of life :

Learning :

1. **Patience:** To be patient is the most valuable asset of life
2. **Perseverance:** learnt not to give up.
3. **Inspiration:** got inspired to become an author by my dad
4. **Happiness:** always live with inner happiness.
5. **Dreams:** Chased my dreams
6. **Forgiveness:** To forgive is to be strong
7. **Myself:** Believe in myself.

Earning :

1. **Goodwill:** the visit was designed to promote relations and goodwill
2. **Love:** loved by friends and family
3. **Friends:** my friends are my pride and are pure souls.
4. **Happiness:** live with self-contentment and inner happiness
5. **Peace:** the state of being calm and quiet in any situation
6. **Devotion:** devotion towards work, God, Self
7. **Aplomb:** became self-confident in demanding situation

Expectation :

1. **Sagacious:** My expectation is to be insightful
2. **Resplendent:** to be shining in an impressive way.
3. **Halcyon:** to remain calm peaceful and carefree.
4. **Ebullient:** Being ebullient will always help me overflow with enthusiasm.
5. **Be Realistic:** can be honest about what you can achieve in a given frame of time.
6. **Accept Change:** will accept change and embrace the uncertainty of life
7. **Allow things to unfold:** when I can find purpose in life if I allow things to unfold.

|| ॐ ||

Deepti Sood

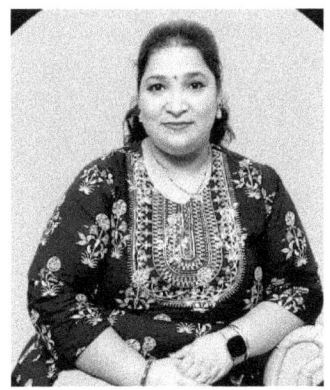

Author's Name	:	Deepti Sood
Qualification	:	Graduate
Current Profession	:	Certified Life Coach & Healer
Age	:	40 years
E-mail ID	:	**ndmmsblogs@gmail.com**
City/ Country	:	**Mumbai, India**

Deepti Sood is a certified life coach, healer, tarot card reader & an influencer. She is passionate about life. Her mission is to help women to discover their life purpose & possibilities to fulfil all their dreams. She served as big sister in a reputed organization and helped more than 100 women's to transform their life journey. She had accomplished her excellence in being Reiki Healer, ho'oponopono healer, crystal healer, aura healer, angel card reader, tarot card reader, A youtuber and an influencer. She is a very loving person who is creative and compassionate about life and is a true fighter. Today she is most grateful for the gift of happiness and gift of gratitude.

The **"Seven LEE of Life"** offers a comprehensive framework for personal and professional development, emphasizing three core areas: **Learning, Earning** and **Expectation.** It advocates for lifelong learning through curiosity and adaptability, strategic earning through diligence and innovation, and balanced expectation management with clarity and patience. This holistic approach encourages continuous self-improvement, financial stability, and realistic goal-setting. By integrating these elements, individuals can navigate life's challenges more effectively, achieve personal and professional success, and maintain a positive, balanced outlook. It's a valuable guide for fostering growth and fulfilment in various aspects of life.

Learning :

1. **Curiosity:** Foster an endless desire to know.
2. **Adaptability:** Embrace change and new methods.
3. **Growth:** Strive for continuous self-improvement.
4. **Insight:** Gain deeper understanding and awareness.
5. **Creativity:** Think outside the box for solutions.
6. **Discipline:** Maintain focus and consistency in learning.
7. **Mindfulness:** Stay present and engaged in the learning process.

Earning :

1. **Strategy:** Plan and execute with purpose.
2. **Persistence:** Keep going despite obstacles.
3. **Savings:** Allocate resources wisely for the future.
4. **Investment:** Grow wealth through smart choices.
5. **Discipline:** Stick to financial plans and budgets.
6. **Adaptability:** Adjust strategies as market conditions change.
7. **Risk Management:** Assess and mitigate financial risks.

Expectation :

1. **Clarity:** Define your goals and desires.
2. **Patience:** Allow time for things to unfold.
3. **Adaptability:** Adjust expectations as new information arises.
4. **Communication:** Express needs and listen to others.
5. **Accountability:** Take responsibility for outcomes.
6. **Boundaries:** Set and respect limits to maintain balance.
7. **Gratitude:** Appreciate progress and small wins.

|| ॐ ||

Divvya A Singh

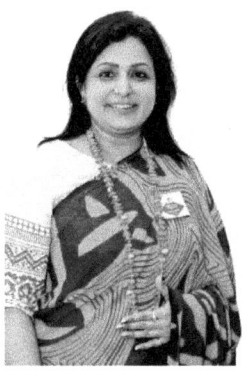

Author's Name	:	Divvya A Singh
Qualification	:	B Sc and B Ed
Current Profession	:	Consultant and Child Coach
Age	:	48 years
E-mail ID	:	**divvyasingh555@gmail.com**
City/ Country	:	**Gurgaon, India**

Divvya A Singh is a Co-founder of Selfwrite Institute of Holistic Development. She is an Educationist and Professional handwriting Analyst, Signature Analyst, Drawing Analyst, Date of Birth Analyst, Hypnotherapist and a Certified Published Author. She has more than 19 years of experience in the teaching sector and 3+ years as a Handwriting Consultant. She is a member of International Council of Graphologist. She is on a mission to empower children and adults and help them nurture their dreams through Graphotherapy, Hypnotherapy and other healing modalities.

'Main zindagi ka saath nibhaata chala gaya

Har fikar ko dhuein mein uraata chala gaya'

- I just keep going with my life, letting each worry fly like smoke..

My life's philosophy mirrors the spirit of this song and I have embraced it fully, living each day in harmony with the message it holds.

'Barbaadiyon ka soz manana fizool tha

Barbaadiyon ka jashn manaata chala gaya'

- It's useless to be unhappy for failing, instead celebrate participation and let go of what can't be controlled.

'Jo mil gaya usi ko muqaddar samajh liya

Jo kho gaya main usko bhulata chala gaya'

- Whatever I get, I take it as my fate and when I lose, I forget it without any remorse.

'Gham aur khushi mein fark na mehsoos ho jahaan

Main dil ko us maqaam pe lata chala gaya'

- Where there is no difference in sorrow and joy, I try to take myself to that point in my heart and soul.

Learning :

1) **Self-Acceptance**: Believing that I'm enough gives me courage to be authentic and an achiever in life.

2) **Celebration:** I celebrate existence and little victories in life by counting smiles but not tears

3) **Surrender:** life is already happening to me, I only enjoy it.

4) **Inner voice**: Inner voice says 'Go for it' - it can be a victory or an experience.

5) **Saying Goodbye**: People teach lessons better than books, so saying good bye doesn't mean I don't like another person, it just means I respect myself too.

6) **Forgiveness**: What other's think of me is none of my business, I always forgives others and myself.

7) **Honesty:** Honesty is an expensive gift, not everyone can afford it.

Earning :

1) **Sanskar:** I am deeply grateful to my proud parents, who instilled the values and teachings in me that makes the backbone of my character and guides me in life and keeps me grounded.

2) **Guru Kripa**: Guru is my guiding light, my unwavering support and the essence of my life's journey, profoundly blessing me with His divine guidance and boundless grace and love.

3) **Jiddu Krishnamurti's philosophy:** My alma mater, under the aegis of Sir Jiddu Krishnamurti's philosophy, provided an environment that deeply influenced my personal growth, helping me evolve into a more thoughtful, self-aware, and compassionate individual.

4) **Purposeful life**: I have co-created peace in my life by practicing mindfulness, and nurturing positive relationships, creating a harmonious and balanced existence for my soul purpose.

5) **God's Grace**: I have embraced the truth that prayer is a highway to God and my life's journey is beautifully graced with His divine presence and blessings.

6) **Eternal love-** I am profoundly touched by the eternal love from my students, whose heartfelt appreciation has always inspired and transformed me into my best version 'A Teacher '

7) **Being Trustworthy**: The unwavering trust from both known and unknown individuals has bestowed upon me the gift of unconditional love and respect in this lifetime, a cherished reward of my journey.

Expectation :

1) **Harmony**: Being in nature teaches us to live in harmony by revealing the delicate balance and interconnectedness of all life forms

2) **Create Heaven**: I create my own heaven with whatever I do, I don't rely on others for my happiness instead cultivate it from within for myself and others.

3) **Be Responsible**: I love my work it satisfies my soul and it's my contribution to the society.

4) **Self-respect**: A lot of people don't deserve my time and it costs me my peace.

5) **Limit Expectation**: Expectation leads to suffering whereas acceptance give us peace and happiness.

6) **Empathy**: we should treat others as we wish to be treated and speak in ways we would be comfortable hearing ourselves, understanding that the other person is just like me a reflection of the same essence that we all share.

7) **Legacy**: I've learned that people will forget what I said or did, but people will never forget how I made them feel. Strive to make a positive impact on others and leave a legacy that reflects our values and contributions as a human being.

॥ ॐ ॥

Courtesty: Song written by Sahir Ludhianvi

Book -Kulliyat-e-Sahir Ludhianvi

Publication-Farid Book Depot (Pvt) Ltd.

Dr A S Poovamma

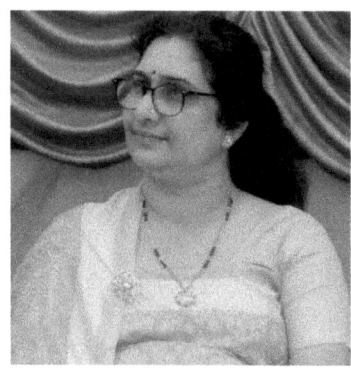

Author's Name	:	Dr. A S Poovamma
Qualification	:	B.AEd. M.A. M.Phil. Ph.D.
Current Profession	:	Rtd. Associate Professor, Former Principal and Vice Principal
Age	:	60 years
E-mail ID	:	…
City/ Country	:	**Gonikoppal, Karnataka, India**

Dr A.S Poovamma now retired from service as an Associate Professor in English in Cauvery College Gonikoppal. She has put in 37 years of service and served as a Lecturer in English, Associate Professor, Head of the Department, Principal and Vice-Principal.

She was the Co-coordinator of IQAC (Internal Quality Assurance Cell) of Cauvery College Gonikoppal in 2010-11 and got Grade 'A' to the institution. She was invited as the Chief-Guest speaker by several institutions and organizations during her long tenure of service. She is a life member of several Literary Associations like MLA, IACLALS, ISPELL. She was the past President of Rotary International organization; Gonikoppal.

She published Poems, Articles, and organized National and International seminars. She also presented papers in National and International Seminars in Hyderabad and in Innsbruck, Austria. She won several Awards like Karnataka Excellence Award in 2021 as the Best Lecturer in English.

'Seven LEE of Life' is a significant topic to think deeply to rejuvenate life in a meaningful way. Compared to other living creatures God has given human life the best of qualities and capacity to use it in a productive manner. But the question is

Is Man using these qualities sensibly? Man is the destroyer of the Universe. If we think sensibly we can generate positive thoughts on **'Seven LEE of Life'**

Learning :

1. **Little Learning:** A little learning is a dangerous thing.
2. **Bread:** Man does not live by bread alone.
3. **Lesson:** Life experience teaches you a great lesson.
4. **Idle Mind:** An Idle Mind is Devil's workshop.
5. **Life:** Life itself is a great Lesson.
6. **Self-help:** Self-Help is the best help.
7. **Too-much:** Too much of anything is harmful.

Earning :

1. **Money:** Earning money is not the only aspect of life though it is important.
2. **Positive Thinking:** We should learn to earn positive thinking to uplift man's life in the human world.
3. **Sacrifice:** One should earn to live well and also to sacrifice.
4. **Donor:** The more you earn, the Great Donor you become.
5. **Experience:** Learn to earn good experience as well so that you can brighten your life and others life as well.
6. **Serve:** Serving the needy is serving God.
7. **Bread:** Man doesn't live by bread alone.

Expectation :

1. **Cleanliness:** Cleanliness is next to Godliness.
2. **Knowledge:** A Little Knowledge is a dangerous thing.
3. **Family:** Family is more sacred than State.
4. **Gold:** Not all that glitters is Gold.
5. **Pen:** Pen is mightier than Sword.
6. **Friend:** A friend in need is a friend indeed.
7. **Race:** Slow and steady wins the race.

॥ ॐ ॥

Dr Agalya VT Raj

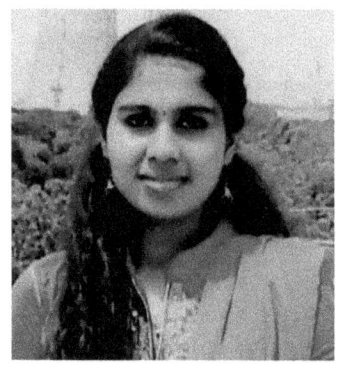

Author's Name	:	Dr. Agalya VT Raj
Qualification	:	M.A., Ph.D. (English)
Current Profession	:	Assistant Professor
Age	:	29 years
E-mail ID	:	**dragalyavtraj@gmail.com**
City/ Country	:	**Chennai, India**

Dr. Agalya VT Raj is an adventurous educator with a passion for communication and teaching. With a Ph.D. in English and a background in teaching and training, she excels in various teaching techniques. Her career spans roles as an Assistant Professor at SRM Institute of Science and Technology. She completed her Doctorate in English at Annamalai University, Chidambaram. Her research is in American Literature. She has published her articles in various Scopus, WOS, UGC Care listed journals and Peer reviewed journals. She has an impeccable writing and editing skills, public speaking, training program management, leadership, curriculum development, project management, and more. Multiple certificates of appreciation and participation in academic and professional development activities, including for NPTEL STAR certifications, NPTEL Translator certifications and international conferences.

'Seven LEE of Life' as an anthology book could symbolize seven pivotal principles or virtues that guide a meaningful existence. "LEE" might be an acronym for essential life elements, such as Love, Empathy, Enlightenment, Leadership, Endurance, Ethics, and Evolution. These principles can encapsulate the human experience, addressing emotional connections, moral integrity, personal growth, and resilience. This anthology might delve into how these themes shape our understanding, interactions, and growth. By weaving diverse perspectives and stories, it would illustrate the interconnectedness of these elements, highlighting their roles in navigating life's complexities. Ultimately, "Seven LEE of Life" can offer readers a comprehensive reflection on the universal and unique aspects of human existence.

Learning:

1) **Love:** Love binds us together and gives meaning to our existence.
2) **Education:** Education empowers individuals and fosters societal progress.
3) **Empathy:** Empathy allows us to understand and connect with others deeply.
4) **Legacy:** Legacy is what we leave behind and how we are remembered.
5) **Evolution:** Evolution drives personal growth and societal advancement.
6) **Endurance:** Endurance helps us overcome challenges and persist through adversity.
7) **Enlightenment:** Enlightenment leads to self-awareness and a deeper understanding of life.

Earning :

1) **Curiosity:** Curiosity drives the quest for knowledge.
2) **Growth:** Growth occurs through continuous learning.
3) **Exploration:** Exploration broadens our understanding of the world.
4) **Adaptation:** Adaptation is essential for survival and progress.
5) **Discovery:** Discovery fuels innovation and creativity.
6) **Reflection:** Reflection enhances the learning process.
7) **Wisdom:** Wisdom is the culmination of lifelong learning.

Expectation :

1) **Work:** Consistent work leads to steady earnings.
2) **Investment:** Smart investments multiply wealth.
3) **Skill:** Developing skills enhances earning potential.
4) **Innovation:** Innovation creates new income opportunities.
5) **Savings:** Savings secure future financial health.
6) **Business:** Running a business can yield significant earnings.
7) **Opportunity:** Seizing opportunities maximizes earnings.

|| ॐ ||

Dr Anisha Mahenrakar

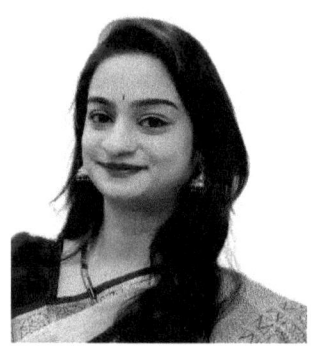

Author's Name	:	Dr. Anisha Mahendrakar
Qualification	:	M.Sc. Counseling Psychology PGDM – Clinical Hypnotherapy, PGDM – Sex Education and Intimacy, 19 Credit Courses –Techniques of Counselling, Methods of Psychological Diagnosis, Asian Healing techniques, PhD
Current Profession	:	Therapist & Healer
Age	:	32 years
E-mail ID	:	**anishamahendrakar@gmail.com**
City/ Country	:	**Bengaluru, India**

Dr. Anisha Mahendrakar is an internationally acclaimed Trainer and Therapist in the field of Psycho-Spiritual wellness. She is renowned for blending traditional values with contemporary techniques and diagnostic tools in psychological counseling. A UNO awardee, Dr. Mahendrakar has been recognized for her outstanding contributions to applied psychology, particularly in managing relationships and intimacy. A child prodigy with a natural talent for tarot card reading and healing, she is also the founder of the Healing modality Rapid Reiki-Quantum Healing. As the founder-director of 'The NewAge Therapist,' a psychological consultancy firm based in Bengaluru, India, Dr. Mahendrakar is dedicated to empowering individuals to blossom into their most authentic selves. She is currently pursuing her second doctorate.

Dr Agalya has the below LEEs of life :

Learning :

1. Patience
2. Art of Speaking
3. Silence
4. Using Intuition
5. The most important things in life are FREE
6. Self Care is First
7. Compassion, when others behave unintelligent.

Earning :

1. Love from People younger than me
2. Respect from people older than me
3. Seeing me as an Inspiration
4. Peace of Mind
5. Self Esteem
6. Self Confidence
7. Self Respect

Expectation :

1. Ethical Behaviour
2. Humane Behaviour
3. Using your Head in business
4. Using your Heart in Relationships
5. Accountability
6. Transparency in Communication
7. Consistency

॥ ॐ ॥

Dr Ellakkiyaa Sankar

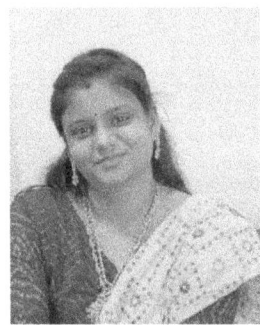

Author's Name	:	Dr. Ellakkiyaa Sankar
Qualification	:	M.A., Ph.D. (English)
Current Profession	:	Assistant Professor in English
Age	:	29 years
E-mail ID	:	**ellakiyashivasankar@gmail.com**
City/ Country	:	**Tamil Nadu, India**

Dr. Ellakkiyaa S is working as Assistant Professor in Erode College of Law, Tamil Nadu. She completed her Doctorate in English in University of Madras. She is a certified Phonic trainer and Handwriting Coach. Her research is on Indian Mythological Fiction. She has published her articles in various UGC Care listed journals, international journals and Peer reviewed journals. She attended 10 seminars, 13 conferences and presented paper in 15 various institutions. She has a better proficiency in English with good grammatical knowledge.

'Seven LEE of Life', denotes the seven learning of human life, which gives a better understanding of thoughts. Gratitude is the key of happiness. When we thank, we get more. A human should be thankful for what he has first. We learn, we experience, we unlearn, we relearn and even after all that we expect something in life. Our expectations should be positive and its turns our life positive. Our thoughts attract the energy around us and attract what we think. We have to have a track of what we learn, we earn and what we expect in our life. While we list what we learn, our confidence level will increase. While we list what we earn, we shall have a satisfaction in our life. While we list what we expect, we will acquire and achieve those through our thoughts.

Learning :

1) Gratitude
2) Self-healing
3) Satisfaction
4) Tolerance
5) Patience
6) I learnt to push myself in hard situations.
7) I learnt to smile.

Earning :

1) My lovable husband
2) Two adorable children
3) Wonderful job
4) Supporting family
5) My doctorate in English
6) My books
7) I am happy for my Chief- Superintendent in my college.

Expectation :

1) Happy Family
2) Healthy and happy Children
3) A Happy family
4) A Successful Entrepreneur
5) A Permanent Job
6) Seven digit earnings in money
7) Fame all over the world

|| ॐ ||

Dr Heena P

Author's Name	:	Dr. Heena P
Qualification	:	AICC, Holistic Healing
Current Profession	:	Consultant and Practitioner
Age	:	50 years
E-mail ID	:	…
City/ Country	:	**New Delhi, India**

Dr. Heena P holds an AICC Certification, demonstrating expertise in holistic health practices. She specializes in: Detoxification and Personalized Weight Loss/ Gain Programs, offering tailored approaches to achieve health goals. Diabetes Reversal Management, providing strategies to manage and potentially reverse diabetes. Support for Lactating Mothers and Pregnancy Nutrition, offering specialized diets to support maternal health and mental health counselling. Sports Nutrition, advising athletes on nutrition to optimize performance. Meditation and Holistic Wellness, certified in AOL Happiness, VTP, DSN and Advance Meditation, Integrating holistic approaches for mental and emotional well-being. Yoga and Meditation Practices, with expertise in BR's Raj Yoga and Holistic Swar Yoga.

Dr. Heena's diverse skills contribute to promoting comprehensive health and well-being through personalized and holistic methodologies.

Dr Heena P has the below LEEs of life :

Learning :

1) **Gita** – The Beautiful Guide to the Journey of Life which taught us to control desires, faith, surrender & detachment from material things.

2) **Learning from Failure** – Failures are the Stepping-stones towards success. Every setback teaches us valuable lessons, helping us to improve & become stronger.

3) **Value Relationship** – They add value to life & create long Lasting happiness that's why we should invest time in building & nurturing these bonds, as they offer support, love & fulfillment.

4) **Power of Kindness** – Being kind fosters positive connections & contributes to a better world. It enhances relationships & inner peace.

5) **Health is Wealth** – Health is the foundation of fulfilling life. Exercise, Proper nutrition & mental wellbeing is necessary to lead a Balanced Life.

6) **Live in Present** – Focusing on present moments allows us to fully appreciate life & reduce anxiety about the past & future.

7) **Embrace Change** – We must learn to adapt & grow with the inevitable changes that come into life. It will bring personal development & opportunities.

These Lessons can guide & motivate us through various phases of Life, offering wisdom & balance.

Earning :

1) **Trust** – Building trust with others is one of the most valuable earnings in one's life. It is earned through honesty, reliability & consistency.

2) **Self-Respect** – Earning it by staying true to our values, maintaining integrity & making choices followed by principles.

3) **Knowledge & Skills** – Lifelong learning & skills are the continuous pursuit of wisdom. It is key earnings that open doors & enrich the mind.

4) **Peace of Mind** – Achievement of peace of mind through forgiveness & letting go of grudges are also considered as earning as it provides priceless emotional balance & happiness.

5) **Karma** – Earning good karma leads us to a better afterlife. It depends on the choices we make.

6) **Legacy** – The impact we leave behind in the form of memories & physical contribution to society represents the lasting earning of our lives.

7) **Face Value** – The person should earn a face value in family and society as well.

These Earnings show the balanced & meaningful approach to living a balanced life.

Expectation :

1) **Happiness** – First & foremost expectation from life is to live with happiness. People seek emotional fulfillment, joy & contentment in life.

2) **Success** – Achieving personal or professional goals whether through career advancement, financial stability or recognition.

3) **Health** – Physical & mental well-being till the end of life.

4) **Growth** – Personal & professional development through learning, new experiences & overcoming challenges.

5) **Security** – Stability in terms of finances, shelter & ability to navigate life's uncertainties with a sense of safety.

6) **Contribution to Society** – Making friends & having social circle, being productive… these all lead us towards the contribution to society as well as maintain harmonious balance in life.

7) **Personal Freedom** – It means financial independence, emotional freedom or freedom from societal pressure which allows us to live life on our own terms.

These Expectations give us hopes, dreams & provide us motivation to move forward without withdrawing.

|| ॐ ||

Dr K G Veena

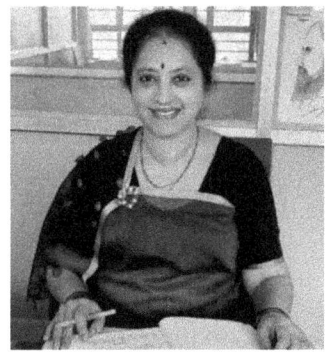

Author's Name	:	Dr. K.G.Veena
Qualification	:	M.A., M.Phil. LL.B., Ph.D.
Current Profession	:	HOD of English, Cauvery College
Age	:	48 years
E-mail ID	:	veenaravindrak@gmail.com
City/ Country	:	Virajpet, Kodagu, India

Dr. K.G.Veena is an academician and a lawyer. She was awarded the doctoral degree from the University of Mysore for her thesis "The Lotus and the Maple: A Comparative Study of the select Novels of Kavery Nambisan and Margaret Atwood. She is presently working as the HOD of English, Cauvery College, Virajpet. She has presented papers in various District, State, National and International Seminars. She has written a few poems and has also translated poems of Kannada and Kodava languages to English. Three of her poems are published. She has edited two books 'Women in Tiger Hills' and 'Inclusion of Kodava Language in the 8th Schedule of Indian Constitution' under the aegis of Karnataka Kodava Sahithiya Academy. She has been a resource person to various talks on 'English Language, Women Rights, Human Rights and in various Legal Awareness programs'.

'Life is Flux' said a famous philosopher named Heraclitus. Life is in a constant state of flux. During our life's span we learn, earn and also expect many things to happen. Life is a great teacher. Life moulds our personality to become refined and eligible to enjoy whatever it bestows on us. A human being is filled with all kinds of emotions such as, happiness, sadness, hatred, jealousy, revenge, disgust, desire, excitement, relief, humour etc., which fills our life with a purpose to live. Life teaches us to nurture commendable feelings and dismiss undeserving and harmful feelings to make our life worth living in this world. Every moment of our life can be made glorious by enhancing learning ability, earning virtues and expecting profound values from the society. Learning, Earning and Expectation must be in tune with living a happy and satisfied life.

Learning:

1. **Lesson**: Life's lesson makes one smarter than before.
2. **Empathy**: To understand and try to solve problems of another.
3. **Ability**: To be able to learn the nuances of life.
4. **Receive**: Learn to receive everything that life offers with humility.
5. **Nicety**: learn the fine and subtle things to bring happiness.
6. **Improve**: Always better ourselves every following day.
7. **Grooming**: Train oneself to face the world with grit and passion.

Earning :

1. **Efficacy**: Being effective to get the desired results.
2. **Admiration**: All seeks to be noticed and admired in this competitive world.
3. **Respect**: Everybody desires to lead a respectful life. Our actions and words decides the respect we earn.
4. **Nobility**: Graciousness captures every mind and heart.
5. **Income:** A decent income would make a comfortable life.
6. **Name**: Good deeds offer respectable name, fame and joy.
7. **Gaiety**: life is all about being happy, so earn cheerfulness wherever you are.

Expectation :

1. **Perfection**: It's a myth! No one and nothing is perfect but can reach near perfection.
2. **Purity:** In this world of blemishes seeking purity is foolishness but can at least expect purity in thoughts.
3. **Wisdom:** Being witty can ease all difficult and problematic situations.
4. **Relaxation:** Never to be a part of the mad rush, so take some time for personal relaxation.
5. **Innocence:** Preserve the child-like innocence to enjoy the creation of God.
6. **Resilience:** Rising and Falling is the norm of life but to bounce back with grace is the sublime attitude.
7. **Fitness:** To be agile and fit until death.

|| ॐ ||

Dr Mahima Mohit Dand

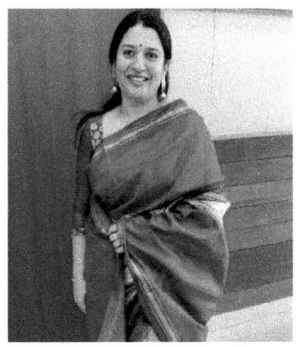

Author's Name	:	Dr. Mahima Mohit Dand
Qualification	:	M.D.S
Current Profession	:	Dentist
Age	:	48 years
E-mail ID	:	mahima702002@yahoo.co.in
City/ Country	:	**Hubli, India**

Dr. Mahima Mohit Dand is a Professor in Conservative Dentistry & Endodontics at SDM Dental College, Dharwad and owns Dr. Mahima's Dentistree in Hubli. A passionate educator, she co-authored a book and contributed to various topics in acclaimed text books, earning her the title of the Most Proactive Academician. She has several publications in national and international journals

An active humanitarian, Dr. Mahima has led impactful service projects as president of Rotary Club of Hubli - Vidyanagar, earning accolades such as Woman of Substance awards in 2021, Best President Award and 12 other honors.

Life is an intricate tapestry woven with experiences, aspirations, and the perpetual journey of self-discovery. Among the myriad facets that shape our existence, three fundamental elements stand out: Learning, Earning and Expectations. These three pillars, collectively known as the **'Seven LEEs of Life',** serve as the cornerstones of personal and professional development. Let me share my personal journey and explore how these elements intertwine to create a fulfilling and balanced life.

'Seven LEE of Life' explores three crucial dimensions: Learning, Earning and Expectations. Each dimension is represented through seven carefully chosen adjectives, providing a nuanced understanding of life's essential components:

Learning :

Learning is the bedrock upon which all progress is built. It is a continuous process that transcends formal education and permeates every aspect of our lives. My journey of learning began at an early age, inspired by my parents, who instilled in me a love for books and curiosity about the world.

1) Continuous
2) Transformative
3) Insightful
4) Dynamic
5) Challenging
6) Engaging
7) Enriching

Earning:

Earning is an essential aspect of life that provides the means to sustain ourselves and fulfill our aspirations. It encompasses not only financial gain but also the broader concept of creating value and contributing to society. While the pursuit of money is often a primary motivator, true earning goes beyond mere monetary compensation.

1) Lucrative
2) Sustainable
3) Rewarding
4) Incremental
5) Substantial
6) Diverse
7) Consistent

Expectation:

Expectations play a pivotal role in shaping our perceptions, aspirations, and interactions. They are the mental frameworks through which we navigate life, influencing our goals, relationships, and overall well-being. Understanding and managing expectations is crucial for achieving a balanced and harmonious life.

1) High
2) Realistic
3) Evolving
4) Achievable
5) Flexible

6) Positive

7) Measured

This collection aims to provide readers with a holistic perspective on personal and professional development, encouraging them to explore, grow and set realistic goals in life.

॥ ॐ ॥

Dr Mehjabeen

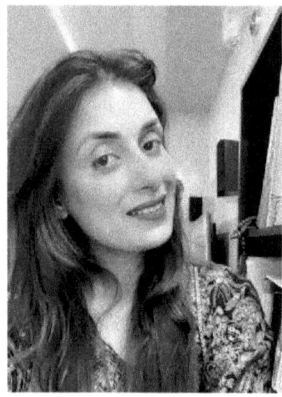

Author's Name	:	Dr. Mehjabeen
Qualification	:	MSc in Clinical Psychology, Doctorate in Psychology
Current Profession	:	Founder of Vision High Mental Wellness, Clinical Psychologist, Psychotherapist, Child Psychologist, Life Coach, Mental Health Ambassador @ Counsel India
Age	:	36 years
E-mail ID	:	mehjabeen7778@gmail.com
City/ Country	:	**Bangalore, India**

Dr Mehjabeen is an accomplished scholar and esteemed author known for her contributions to journal related to Mental Health and other helpful topics, which can make a huge difference in other lives. She has authored numerous publications that have significantly impacted relevant disciplines, where she has also been involved in ground breaking research. Her work is characterized by a commitment to specific themes, values or methodologies, making her a respected voice in her field. In addition to her academic pursuits, Dr Mehjabeen is actively engaged in such as community service contributions towards mental health public speaking, journaling further showcasing her dedication to advancing knowledge and fostering positive change.

Dr. Mehjabeen is a distinguished psychologist and the visionary founder of Vision High Mental Wellness. with an extensive background in psychology, she has dedicated her career to promoting mental health and well-being.

This anthology not only provides insightful reflections and practical advice, but also inspires readers to reflect on their own journeys and make conscious efforts to enrich their lives. Embracing the **'Seven LEE of Life'** paves the way for personal growth, happiness and a deeply satisfying life. Each chapter delves into a core principle—Learning, Earning, Expectation, Responsibility, Balance, Gratitude and Fulfillment—offering both philosophical insights, set realistic goals, take accountability, maintain harmony, appreciate life's blessings, and seek purpose. These principles are interwoven by embracing these **'LEEs'**, readers are encouraged to foster a lifelong passion for knowledge, cultivate financial and emotional resilience, set and manage realistic expectations, uphold responsibilities with integrity, find harmony between life's demands, practice gratitude and seek genuine fulfillment. This anthology is a call to action, urging readers to consciously integrate these values into their lives, thereby creating a more enriched, purposeful and joyful existence.

'Seven LEE of Life' invites you to embark on a transformative journey toward becoming the best version of yourself.

Learning :

1. Curiosity: The foundation of all knowledge.

2. Growth: Embrace every opportunity to expand your mind.

3. Persistence: Keep learning despite obstacles.

4. Reflection: Learn from past experiences.

5. Adaptability: Be open to new ways of thinking.

6. Inquiry: Always ask questions and seek answers.

7. Wisdom: Apply what you've learned to make better decisions.

Earning :

1. Income: The result of hard work.

2. Skill: Develop valuable abilities to increase earning potential.

3. Opportunity: Seek out chances to advance financially.

4. Investment: Use earnings wisely to grow wealth.

5. Balance: Find a healthy balance between work and life.

6. Gratitude: Appreciate the fruits of your destiny.

7. Impact: Use your gratitude to make a positive difference.

Expectation :

1. Hope: The driving force behind aspirations.

2. Realism: Balance dreams with practicality.

3. Patience: Good things take time.

4. Clarity: Be clear about what you expect from life.

5. Flexibility: Be willing to accept expectations.

6. Choice: Choose wisely your choices and not to blame on your destiny.

7. Fulfillment: Achieve contentment by aligning expectations with reality.

॥ ॐ ॥

Dr Navjot Kaur

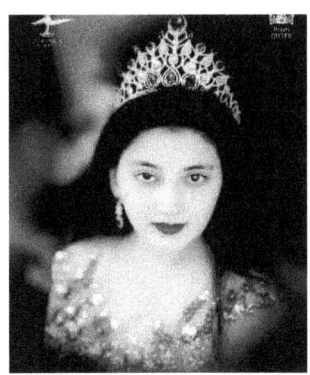

Author's Name	:	Dr. Navjot Kaur
Qualification	:	M.B.A., Ph.D. (Management)
Current Profession	:	Educationist
Age	:	31 years
E-mail ID	:	**drnavjotkaur29@gmail.com**
City/ Country	:	**Vancouver, Canada**

Dr. Navjot Kaur, is a young dynamic educationist. She is a Director of Administration of an eminent educational institution and an active member of the Advisory Board to schools. Adorning several crowns, she is a true beauty with purpose, an educationist by profession with the fundamental aim to enlighten several lives. She believes in imparting right knowledge and encouraging women to believe in their dreams and unleash one's true potential.

She received numerous international and national accolades and awards for exemplary leadership skills in the field of education. She is a woman with power and positive influence, who exudes unprecedented strength and valour with optimistic outlook to face all challenges of life tenaciously.

Dr Navjot Kaur is a truly epitome of beauty with brain as winning the national title of Mrs. India Planet 2022. She proved to be an inspiration and encouragement to ample of women to believe in themselves and vanquish greatness in life. With a vibrant blend of grace, intellect, and dedication, Dr. Navjot Kaur has made her mark, embodying the true spirit of an empowered and inspirational woman.

'Seven LEE of life' as deciphered stands for seven Learnings Earnings and Expectations of life. These are the inter-related aspects of our life that shape our persona and influence our growth.

Learning is a lifetime endeavor that encompasses the principle, ethics and values leading us to be the best versions of ourselves.

Earning is an intangible outcome of learning. Earnings of life comprises of blessings, wisdom, love, respect, serenity in behavior. These all are the phenomenal aspects of real earnings in an individual's life. Earning in life isn't just about accumulating financial wealth, imperatively it is about acquiring and appreciating the true blessings that contribute to a dignified and fulfilling existence.

Expectations from life and ourselves arise from experiences, right knowledge and wisdom. Life experiences and memories are priceless. Exploring new places, acquiring knowledge, and creating memories with family and friends add value to life that goes beyond material belongings.

Learning:

1. **Compassion:** Being kind & compassionate is a virtue, the ability to comprehend and empathize with the emotions of others is important.

2. **Courage:** Embracing one's true self and expressing ideas and believes valiantly fosters self-worth.

3. **Resilience:** Developing the ability to bounce back from setbacks and face challenges with a positive mindset.

4. **Gratitude:** Practicing thankfulness, extending gratitude can help us see the blessings in our life.

5. **Forgiveness:** Forgiveness is the act of letting go of resentment, anger, or the desire for vengeance. Forgiveness immensely allows us to move past negative emotions and promotes inner peace.

6. **Making every Moment Count:** Time is the most precious resource, and it's limited, live life to the fullest making every moment count.

7. **Responsibility:** Being responsible fosters personal growth, better relationships, builds integrity and leads to success.

Earning:

1. **Spiritual Discipline:** The activities and practices that support one's inner life and connection to a higher power, moral principles, or more profound sense of purpose develops spiritual consciousness.

2. **Love:** Love is the biggest earning in life. Love in all forms-be it the love of your parents, family or self-love enriches our lives in ways that materialistic things can't buy.

3. **Respect:** Authenticity is the bedrock of earnings it develops true respect in the hearts of others.

4. **Blessings:** The most precious gift that can be given and an individual's real earning is true blessings. Acknowledging blessings in our life fosters happiness.

5. **Knowledge and Wisdom:** Right knowledge is information whereas wisdom is applying that knowledge at the right time and situations. Knowledge empowers us and wisdom opens new horizons.

6. **Noble Karma:** "What goes around, comes around", Noble karma rooted in good deeds, creates a cycle of positive energy.

7. **Moral Fiber:** Having a strong ethical fiber is a sheer blessing in an individual's life.

Expectation:

1. **Contentment:** The significant expectation from life is to be happy and spread joy around. Contentment unlocks doors of achievement and success.

2. **Exploring to the World:** Travelling is an opportunity to new experiences and embrace the beauty of this earth.

3. **Health and Well-Being:** Investing in health through a balanced lifestyle is immensely imperative. Positive mental health equips with resilience to bounce back even stronger from the setbacks of life.

4. **Freedom:** The ability to make choices and have control over one's life is a key expectation. This includes the freedom to pursue one's passions, make personal decisions, and live according to one's values and beliefs.

5. **Constant Learning:** Investing time and energy in learning, upskilling own abilities and talents leads to vanquishing greatness in life.

6. **Adhere to the path of righteousness:** Being righteous, taking responsibility for one's actions and walking on the path of truthfulness.

7. **Leading an Inspirational life:** A life dedicated in imparting right knowledge to children and inspiring women to invest in their skills and unleash their hidden potential to achieve their goals.

I hope my opinion encourages others to pursue their own aspirations, to experience the world and to cherish every moment. Let my legacy be one of inspiration, showing that with dedication and love, anything is possible.

|| ॐ ||

Dr Noothan Rao

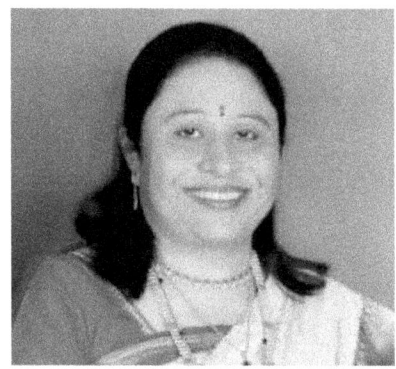

Author's Name	:	Dr. Noothan Rao
Qualification	:	B.Com, Doctorate.
Current Profession	:	Counselor, Astrologer & Graphologist
Age	:	52 years
E-mail ID	:	**noothan.wswrt@gmail.com**
City/ Country	:	**Bengaluru, India**

Dr. Noothan Rao- Counsellor, Graphologist. Formerly working for Canara Bank, currently involved in activities of integrated, holistic healing at *"Write Strokes with Right Thoughts™"*, *Research Center, based in Bengaluru, India, offering services across globe.*

Professional qualifications: B.Com, ICWAI – Inter, Internationally Certified Handwriting analyst & Grapho-analytical Therapist, Certified Personal Counselor & Company Director, Doctorate & Professorship in Astrology, Honorary Doctorate in Advanced Graphology. Many more certificates in various Healing modalities. Presented papers at **National Women's Science Congress,** won best paper award & **Woman Scientist** award.

She trains people in personality development, goal setting, vision, Career guidance, Handwriting analysis, Grapho therapy and Art analysis to understand self/others. She is also working on various other interests of hers in the field of Counseling, Astrology, Tarot Reading, Dowsing Geopathic stress removal. She is giving integrated therapy to cure many medical problems. Her articles on all these areas are published in various websites, magazines, and Social Medias. Her interview has come in FM Rainbow (AIR India) under inspire program, California Radio etc. She has been called by TV for expert opinion on subjects.

Most people don't like advices, suggestions. Somewhere it feels like criticism or pinpointing their lack of abilities to lead life. There again body language, tonality, attitude of the advisor affects a lot. Relationship ego also comes into picture. They don't see the content & its validity. They just think who is he/she to say that to me?

People get inspired or influenced by real life stories/experiences. When it is in the form of book/documentary/video/movie - people get that freedom of choosing the subject to take and apply. No one is forcing them to do anything there.

It's a wonderful idea to come up with Anthology book wherein so many people write their life story, understandings, learnings, failures, success stories. Future generations can benefit from this non-intrusive method of support.

It also gives an opportunity for so many people to share their experiences and viewpoint on the topic. It's a creative expression of their feelings and emotions. It brings out their writing skill, gives exposure to whole new world.

'Seven LEE of Life' is one such attempt to brin gout all those life experiences in pointers to ponder. This is my insight into the topic:

Learning :

1) Is experiential & lifelong.
2) Removes boredom.
3) Learn by exploring places and reading books.
4) Prodigies are born because our soul carries the learning to next life.
5) Makes us unique, special, popular and successful.
6) Learn to let go.
7) Learn to share and grow.

Earning :

1) Earn while learning.
2) Earn name, fame, money, love, respect, blessings, happiness, trust.
3) Successful people are remembered, hence earn to become successful.
4) Money is important, take responsibility of it.
5) Earning through the right method gives peace and satisfaction.
6) Equally distributed wealth to all is **Time,** Earn & use it wisely.
7) Correct your frequency & belief system about earning.

Expectation :

1) Expectation is natural as long as we are alive.

2) All living beings expect one or the other things always.

3) Don't expect to change others unless they are willing.

4) Expecting the unexpected brings constant anticipation & anxiety.

5) Determination leads to meet self and other's expectations.

6) Doing what is "Inspected" not what is "expected" is deceit.

7) Expect your desire to be fulfilled yet detach from outcome.

॥ ॐ ॥

Dr Priti Doshi

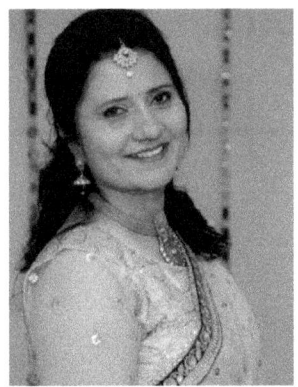

Author's Name	:	Dr. Priti Doshi
Qualification	:	PhD in Numerology
Current Profession	:	Healer and Professional Teacher of Occult Sciences
Age	:	49 years
Email ID	:	**pritidoshi809@gmail.com**
City/ Country	:	**Mumbai, India**

Dr. Priti Doshi is a certified numerologist, tarot card reader, astrologer and a diploma holder in graphology. She has various modalities to share and to recount a part of her personal life journey, how she was and motivated towards this profession. It is truly said that difficult times make you stronger. When she was 15, her father was retired, since he was an only medium of the financial securities. She took up an opportunity to support the family at the age of 15 years and sacrificed her dream to become a doctor since she wished her younger brother to study well.

Priti Doshi opted for B.Com. instead of pursuing her dream of becoming a Doctor. After working hard, She cleared B.Com, and got married and became a mother of two. Despite financial challenges, she began giving tuitions at 15, continuing for over 30 years, eventually becoming a proficient phonics and grammar teacher. Facing Vastu dosh in her new house, She started the journey in the occult sciences to heal her home and family members. For the past nine years, she has been constantly helping others as a professional tarot card reader, numerologist and astrologer.

I have a deep appreciation for meaningful and insightful literature about **"Seven Lee,"** this anthology book explores themes of personal growth, spirituality and the balance between learning, earning and expectations. This could include stories, essays, and reflections on the diverse ways people think and their achievements about financial stability and success. It might explore the challenges and triumphs of different professions, the impact of economic conditions, and personal anecdotes of financial growth it can be about the pursuit of knowledge and personal development. Contributions might range from academic achievements and lifelong learning journeys to the role of education in shaping one's future. And expectations may have hopes, goals and aspirations that drive individuals.

Learning :

1) **Never trust anyone blindly:** It's important to be discerning and thoughtful in our relationships and decisions.

2) **Always listen to your parents:** Parents often have valuable life experiences and wisdom to share.

3) **Listen to the universal message:** Being attuned to the greater truths and messages around us can guide us on our path.

4) **Have strong bonding with your children:** Building a close relationship with your children fosters love, trust, and mutual respect.

5) **Work to bring a smile to others' faces daily:** Small acts of kindness can make a big difference in someone's day.

6) **Always do your activity as a pure soul:** Acting with integrity and purity of heart brings peace and fulfillment.

7) **Always support everyone:** Offering support and encouragement helps build a stronger, more compassionate community.

Earning :

1) **Self-made person:** I have built my life and success through my own efforts and determination.

2) **With my family:** I am the pillar of support and love for my family.

3) **Wonderful mother:** I nurture and guide my children with unconditional love and wisdom.

4) **Build good relationships in family:** I foster harmony and strong bonds within my family.

5) **Have a good number of friends:** I cherish and maintain meaningful friendships.

6) **Spiritual advisor:** I guide others on their spiritual journeys with insight and compassion.

7) **Very good teacher:** I inspire and educate my students with passion and dedication.

Expectation :

1) **I want to leave the world peacefully:** Striving for inner peace and harmony can help you achieve this goal.

2) **I don't want people to cry after I leave:** It's touching that you care so much about the well-being of others, even after you're gone.

3) **I believe whatever I do; I do it selflessly:** Acting with selflessness is a noble trait that can inspire others.

4) **People have grown materialistic:** It's true that materialism can overshadow deeper values, but your perspective can help remind others of what truly matters.

5) **I have always stood for everyone selflessly:** Your dedication to supporting others is commendable and likely appreciated by many.

6) **People remember me for my good deeds:** Leaving a legacy of kindness and good deeds is a beautiful way to be remembered.

7) **If my name can bring a smile on their face:** Bringing joy to others through your actions and memory is a wonderful aspiration.

|| ॐ ||

Dr Priyadarshini MM

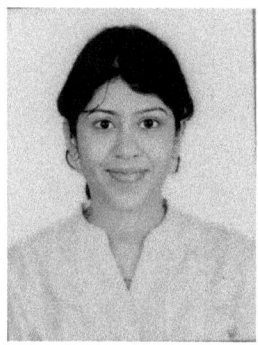

Author's Name	:	Dr. Priyadarshini MM
Qualification	:	MBBS, MD
Current Profession	:	Associate Professor Pathology
Age	:	39 years
E-mail ID	:	**log2piya@gmail.com**
City/ Country	:	**Kodagu India**

Kodavathi, Doctor by profession, Pathologist working as Associate Professor at the pristine Kodagu Institute of Medical Sciences nestled in a small Hill station, Kodagu, Karnataka. Took to poetry and writing after getting influenced by her Mother quoting William Wordsworth who said "Poetry is the spontaneous overflow of powerful feelings: it takes its origin from emotion recollected in tranquility". Writing and poetry came naturally during her moments of travel. Found solace in placing emotions on to words! Being a Doctor she has managed to create a perfect space to blend creativity and writing and has a Poetry book named 'Soul Baggage'- poetic captures of emotions.

Dr Priyadarshini has the below LEEs of life :

Learning :

1) From wise words
2) Profound Phrases
3) Stimulating Sentence
4) Poignant Paragraph
5) Powerful Pages

6) Comprehensive Chapters

7) To a bounteous Book

Earning :

1) Zillion Smile

2) Being an Inspiration

3) Self improvement

4) Radiate cheer

5) Gain insights

6) Wide spread Knowledge

7) Self confidence

Expectation :

1) Content heart

2) Happy mind

3) Self motivation

4) Clarity on confusion

5) Positive Impact

6) Unwind the mind

7) Critical acclaim

|| ॐ ||

Dr Shalini Garg

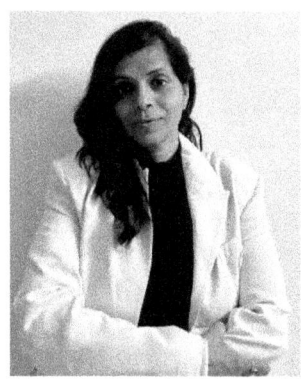

Author's Name	:	Dr. Shalini Garg
Qualification	:	Ph.D. in Psychology
Current Profession	:	Life Coach and Healer
Age	:	49 years
E-mail ID	:	**shalinigarg630@gmail.com**
City/ Country	:	**Alwar (Rajasthan), India**

Dr. Shalini Garg is a dedicated educator with a lifelong passion for teaching and learning. She completed her schooling at a convent in Delhi and graduated from Delhi University. She started her career as a computer teacher at a very young age of 19yrs.

After marriage, she had to take a long career break due to family expectations. However, she continued her academic journey, earning a Ph.D. in Psychoanalysis and later working as an English Professor.

Dr. Shalini Garg has authored two books that are soon to be published and she regularly writes blogs on Medium. Love writing poems that reflect her creativity.

She has also published research papers in UGC CARE-listed journals.

During the pandemic, she discovered life skills courses that provided essential tools for coping with the emotional challenges of the time. Inspired by the knowledge she learned from leading coaches and today she's a certified life coach, graphotherapist, Reiki healer and an inner child healer. She offers free online healing sessions as a part of her service to humanity. Her mission is to raise awareness and encourage people to take responsibility for everything happening in their lives, as all change begins within. She believes, change the perspective and the world around you will automatically change.

The anthology **'Seven LEE of Life'**, featuring 108 writers, promises to be an extraordinary experience for readers. With such a vast number of contributors each offering their unique take on the Seven LEEs — where L stands for Learning, E for Earning and E for Expectation — readers will get a lot of inputs and clarity.

In the first **L** the learnings shared by the authors are personal and deeply reflective, shaped by the experiences that define their lives. These are learnings that cannot be taught in classrooms but are acquired through life's trials and triumphs.

The **E** of earnings, in this context, transcend financial wealth and touch upon the true riches of life—knowledge, wisdom, love, contribution, and service. These are the intangible assets that not only enhance one's current existence but also leave behind a legacy for future generations.

The third aspect **E** for expectations, is equally significant, as it reveals what each individual hopes for—whether from society, from loved ones, or from life itself. These expectations are unique to every person, shaped by their journey and inner growth.

This anthology will undoubtedly inspire readers to reflect on their own LEEs offering perspectives that could guide them in their own journeys.

Learning:

1. **Connection with the Source:** Cherish and resolve conflicts with our parents, as they are the foundation of our existence.
2. **Self-Love:** Cultivate self-love and care for our overall well-being, instead of seeking external validation.
3. **Gratitude:** Embrace gratitude as a vital practice by regularly acknowledging and counting our blessings.
4. **Forgiveness:** Let go of past hurts by forgiving others and seeking forgiveness, a path to inner peace and emotional healing.
5. **Live in the Present:** Focus on the present moment, as it is the only time we truly have to make the most of life.
6. **Balanced Perspective:** Accept both good and bad as a part of life and maintain a balanced outlook.
7. **Service and Contribution:** Engage in acts of service to help the underprivileged, nurturing empathy and compassion for others.

Earnings :

1. **My Loved Ones:** My family, friends, and loved ones are my most valuable assets, providing love and lasting bonds I will always cherish.
2. **Education:** My education defines who I am and will continue to inspire and serve me throughout my life.

3. **Gratitude:** The realization of my blessings brings abundance, and practicing gratitude enriches every aspect of life.
4. **Knowledge, Wisdom, and Degrees:** The wisdom from my mentors and the degrees I've earned, PhD, Life Coaching, Graphology, Healing etc. give me a sense of pride and a purpose to contribute to the society.
5. **My Creativity:** My ability to express myself through poems, blogs, and books is a treasured gift.
6. **Compassion and Empathy:** I feel blessed to have compassion for the needy and a genuine desire to help.
7. **Knowledge of Self and Spirituality:** Understanding that I am pure consciousness, connected to a higher eternal power, guides me toward unity and oneness with all.

Expectations :

1. **Take Responsibility:** I expect everyone needs to take responsibility for their lives instead of blaming others.
2. **Let Go:** People should release mental clutter and let go of things that negatively impact their well-being and relationships.
3. **Invest in You:** I encourage my loved ones and society to invest in personal growth and continuous learning beyond formal education.
4. **Don't Judge:** I want people to avoid judging others and instead focus on self-reflection and introspection.
5. **Be Authentic:** I value authenticity and transparency, and I wish for my loved ones to avoid fake attitudes.
6. **Respect and Acknowledgment:** I expect respect and recognition for the effort I put into my writing and coaching.
7. **Fame and Recognition:** I aim to achieve global success and recognition in my writing and coaching journey.

॥ ॐ ॥

Giresh LD Chawda

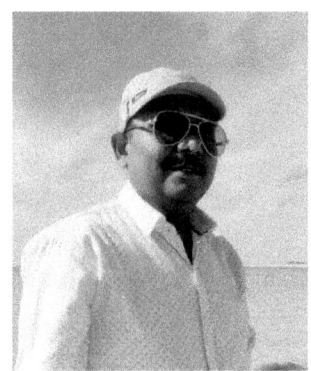

Author's Name	:	Giresh LD Chawda
Qualification	:	B.Com, Computer Hardware & Networking Engineer
Current Profession	:	Graphic Designer, Creative Artist
Age	:	42 years
E-mail ID	:	**gireshldchawda@gmail.com**
City/ Country	:	**Indore, India**

Giresh LD Chawda mainly belongs to the cleanest city of India, Indore MP. He has completed his graduation in Commerce and during his graduation, he completed his Diploma in Computer Hardware and Networking.

But as per his destiny, he is doing his ancestral printing work, which was being done by the previous generations as per the current new format and trend as the third generation, for this he has done Diploma in Graphic Designing along with printing and advertising as well. Having received training and certification, he has worked for many Corporate & reputed spiritual institutions, in Simhastha 2015 he worked for Namami Gange project in Ujjain, in 2018, done branding for IPL matches in Indore. He is providing advertising and printing services in his city as well as all over India as the director of Yash Enterprise,

Simultaneously, Giresh has a deep interest in the spiritual field, during pandemic period and lockdown, he studied Numerology and got certified training in Reiki and Marma Chikitsa for public welfare.

'**Seven LEE of Life**' is a very interesting and difficult topic in itself, it is not so easy to say and write on this topic because each and every word will become a source of inspiration for many people. The work done by Rainu Mangatani Ma'am of first finding 108 pearls in the form of teachers from around the world and then weaving them all into one thread through Abhishaik Chitraans Sir, compiler of our book under the inspiration of God, is highly appreciated... The joint effort of all of 108 co-authers will definitely give a new experience to our readers and will blossom the seeds of innovation in everybody's life.

Learning :

1. Our life neither in the past nor in the future, only the proper utilization of the present time becomes the medium for innovation of new life.

2. Whether you are 6 years old or 60 years old, you should always continue learning in life, because this skill gives you unique fuel to live life.

3. Whenever you feel disappointment or frustration, start increasing your contact with nature and whatever situation you are in at present, try to spend time with people who are one notch below your level, everything else will automatically go up in smoke.

4. Do not forget the most bitter time of your life because it was the one that laid the foundation for living every joy and happiness that came later.

5. The real shelter of God is experienced only when, before asking for forgiveness for our sins, we forgive others in our thoughts, words and deeds - seek their forgiveness and worship to God.

6. Those with whom we have close relations in our life should not waste our energy on improving more than necessary after making proper efforts and not getting results. After some time they emerge as our biggest enemies.

7. We should find a Guru in our life only after searching, thinking and examining, who can be the guide for the progress and salvation of our soul in the present life, without any deceit or selfishness.

I agree that there is a lot of pain in our relationships in our lives, but I also know that it is possible to overcome the deeds of one's own previous births in the present birth only on the basis of spiritual knowledge and its learning & proper implementation on each path of life.

Earning :

1. Learn and teach how to earn blessings more than once every day with your skills, cooperation and courage.

2. In the hustle and bustle of everyday life, one should make some small efforts for the other so that both of them feel happy, do not try too much with those who are not worthy of it. Otherwise you will get the opposite result.

3. For the progress of our soul along with the body, one must practice any Sattvik medium like worship, meditation and study of spiritual books that are easily accepted.

4. We should try to help the elderly, lonely and destitute people through our thoughts, words and deeds to the best of our ability. This effort becomes a medium of unforgettable and invaluable blessings in your life.

5. Our souls' spiritual happiness can never be bought on the basis of money, for this one has to forget one's own existence and experience it on the ladder of blessings and without any expectations towards God.

6. We fought the entire universe after being born in this human life, the miracle of the 21st century has made us forget even God, has erased all our feelings of belongingness and has entangled us in a maze, give a break to your mind, because even God must be saying that you have forgotten me in the web of illusion, the hell of Kaliyuga.

7. Apart from our education & common knowledge, we should study the divine virtues for our soul and understand them from our Vedas, Puranas and spiritual interpretations and make every effort to imbibe them in our present life because these earnings remain with us even after we leave this world.

Expectation :

1. I request the Universe to open such a hospital in which treatment of any kind of disease can be imparted through various mediums like Naturopathy, Healing, Reiki, Marma Therapy, Neurotherapy, Panchakarma along with teaching how to live life with spiritual values.

2. In this world, hypocrisy, opportunism, giving pain or hurting someone through thoughts, words and deeds, this happens to many people, but after experiencing all these, we have to save ourselves, in this the Satvik spiritual path helps us a lot & Gives guidance.

3. With the help of the Supreme Father, Supreme Soul and Gurus, I meet in my life. I wish to see my coming life reach such a stage that I can be become the best medium for the welfare of other living beings through the spiritual teachings and experience gained from them.

4. Whenever we sit before God, we should go with the same feeling as if we meet a VIP of this world at the appointed time, with full heart and happiness. When we approach God, the most VVIP of the world, through worship, prayer and meditation, we too leave aside the thoughts, sorrows and thoughts going on in our lives and become completely empty-headed and happy feelings. And you should come face to face with great enthusiasm, then the experience will inspire you to live your life out of the box way.

5. Pray to God, this book has written a unique treatise in yourself which will become the lifeline of the spirit somewhere in the world. Our books will carve out a unique place for you in the world and prove to be a unique best seller.

6. We have come here as an inheritance with many unique gifts like unique nature and divine virtues which are our keys in life which we are presented with by the universe for our future. Our gurus always give us the opportunity to take a dip in the glory of our divine virtues. Here's a prayer for soul welfare

7. Thanks to the universe that I was also selected among 108 writers and provided a new opportunity to express my ideas in life and with the same aspiration that I will get opportunities in the future also.

|| ॐ ||

Harishita

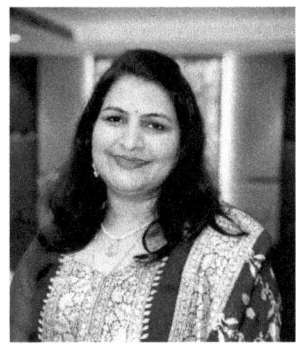

Author's Name	:	Harishita (Vicky Chauhan)
Qualification	:	B.P.Ed., M.A. in Yoga
		Diploma in Acupressure, Diploma in Neurotherapy
Current Profession	:	Life Coach, Counselor, Energy Healer
Age	:	41 years
E-mail ID	:	**harishita10@gmail.com**
City/ Country	:	**Noida, India**

Harishita, CEO and Founder of **Sacred Healing**, The Institute of Energy Healing, Occult Sciences and Research having global certification and recognition ie. ISO 9001:2015, She is a multifaceted healer and therapist with expertise in various modalities. Her specialties include Energy Healing: Focusing on balancing and restoring the body's energetic fields for improved physical, emotional and spiritual health. Mokshapatta Reading: Utilizing the ancient Indian board game for spiritual guidance and self-awareness. Tarot Card Reading: Providing insight and clarity through tarot, a tool for personal growth and decision-making. Neurotherapy: Addressing neurological issues by regulating the nervous system. Sound Healing: Using vibrational sound to promote deep relaxation and healing. Life Coaching: Guiding individuals toward achieving their personal and professional goals through holistic support.

Harishita's work integrates these practices to help clients achieve balance and well-being on multiple levels. She has experience of 15 Years in this field.

In this book, one will read life perspectives of 108 Co-authors. By which one can get better understanding of life. One can get a great amount of knowledge and different perspectives in just a single book. So, a person can correct their way of living life. I thank Mr. Abhishaik Chitraans for giving this opportunity.

Learning :

1. **Curiosity** – Sparks the pursuit of new knowledge and experiences.
2. **Awareness** – Expands understanding of ourselves and the world.
3. **Adaptability** – Enables us to embrace change and evolve.
4. **Challenge** – Overcoming obstacles strengthens resilience and wisdom.
5. **Reflection** – Helps in understanding past experiences for better decision-making.
6. **Perseverance** – Sustains us through challenges and setbacks.
7. **Patience** – Essential for the gradual unfolding of meaningful learning.

Earning :

1. **Discipline** – Consistent effort is key to sustainable earning.
2. **Value** – Providing value drives long-term success and rewards.
3. **Skill** – Mastery of skills increases earning potential.
4. **Persistence** – Overcoming setbacks is essential for financial stability.
5. **Balance** – Managing family and work ensures well-rounded wealth.
6. **Trust** – Earned trust in my career life.
7. **Love** – Earned love of my family and clients. Earning love and trust is the most important thing for life.

Expectation :

1. **Hope** – Expectations often stem from a sense of optimism.
2. **Patience** – Managing expectations requires the virtue of waiting.
3. **Adaptability** – Flexibility allows expectations to evolve with circumstances.
4. **Trust** – Expectations often rely on faith in others or outcomes.
5. **Growth** – Adjusting expectations fosters personal development.
6. **Attachment** – Strong expectations can lead to emotional dependence. Don't get so attached to someone. Don't expect anything from anyone because if we expect and our expectations are broke. It gives immense pain, sometimes which we can't even handle.
7. **Acceptance** – Embracing outcomes helps in overcoming unmet expectations.

|| ॐ ||

Harsatvir Kaur

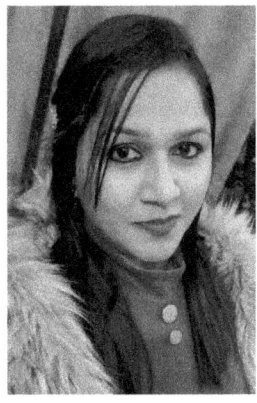

Author's Name	:	Harsatvir Kaur
Qualification	:	M.A. (History), B.Ed.
Current Profession	:	Teacher
Age	:	36 years
E-mail ID	:	...
City/ Country	:	**Mohali, India**

Harsatvir Kaur is a teacher, who has done her Bachelor Degree in Arts and Master Degree in History. After that she has done her Bachelor of Education Degree with Punjabi and SST subjects. She has also cleared the Teacher Eligibility Test. She has four years' experience in teaching. She has won many zonal and state level prices in co-curricular activates. Along with reading and teaching she also enjoys writing. And so, fourth slowly, she also works to put pearls of words in sentences. She is now budding author.

Dear Readers, I would like to share some words about this anthology book. First of all I would like to tell you that how I came to know about this book. Actually, my mother who has been the student of Abhishaik Sir, told about his commendable work. After discussion with my husband, I contacted Abhishaik Sir to become the part of this book.

Dear Readers through this book we will get to know about the three different aspects of life which are co-related with each other, these aspects are learning, earning and expectation. They play most important role in everyone life. Learning is a continuous process as we always learn something in every moment in our life. Similarly we always expected something in our life every day. Like this earning is also the most important part of our life.

Learning :

1. **Growth:** Learning is something we do throughout our lives to help us grow and improve.
2. **Problem Solving:** It helps us to think better and solve problems we face every day.
3. **Uunderstanding:** By learning new things, we understand more about the world and how it works.
4. **Creativity:** It also encourages us to be creative and come up with new ideas
5. **Learning** teaches us to keep going even when things are hard.
6. **Useful:** In today's world, it is important to keep learning so we can stay up to date and be useful in personal and professional lives.
7. **Better Being:** In the end learning helps us become better people and make a positive difference.

Earning :

1. Earning is important because it provides the means to support ourselves and our families.
2. It allows us to meet essential needs like food, housing and healthcare.
3. Future Saving: Through earning we can save for the future and handle unexpected expenses.
4. Freedom: It also gives us the freedom to make choices such as investing in education or perusing personal goals.
5. Having a steady income contributes to a sense pf security and wellbeing.
6. Ultimately, earning is the key to building a stable and fulfilling life.
7. Earning is good to live, but it is not everything to live.

Expectation :

1. **Hope:** Expectations are beliefs or hopes about what will happen in the future.
2. **Guidance:** They guide how we approach situations and relationships, shaping our thought and actions
3. **Motivation:** Having clear expectations can help to set goals and motives us to achieve them.
4. **Sometimes Disappointment:** However, unrealistic expectation can lead to disappointment if things don't turn as we hoped.
5. **Balance:** It is important to balance optimism with a realistic outlook.
6. **Interactions:** Expectations also affect how we interact with others, as we may expect certain behaviour out comes from them.
7. **Satisfaction:** Managing expectations well can lead to greater satisfaction and better relationship.

In the end I would like to the entire team who consider me worthy of this . Hope you find this Anthology Book close to your heart.

॥ ॐ ॥

Himani Bajaj

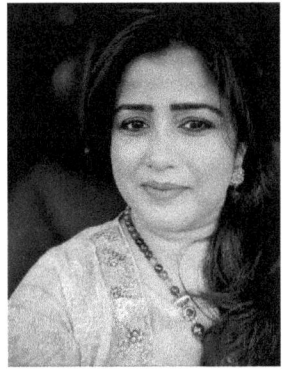

Author's Name:	:	Himani Bajaj
Qualification:	:	B.Tech. Computer Engineering, Harmonized Life License Qualification
Current Profession:	:	Entrepreneur, Financial Advisor, Occult Science Practitioner, AP with SKY Kundalini
Age:	:	47 years
E-mail ID:	:	**bajajhimani@gmail.com**
City/ Country:	:	**Toronto, Canada**

Himani Bajaj is an accomplished entrepreneur with over 15 years of experience in the financial industry. She is dedicated to empowering families through a deep understanding of financial concepts. Holding a B. Tech in Computer Engineering, she combines her technical expertise with financial insight to offer valuable guidance to her clients.

Himani emphasizes the importance of both financial and mental health, recognizing how much numbers can influence individuals and their decisions. She helps her clients make better choices in every aspect of their lives.

In addition to her work in finance, Himani is a Certified Numerologist and Vastu specialist/ consultant. She also serves as an assistant professor specializing in Simplified Kundalini Yoga (SKY) in Canada. SKY is an Integrated Wellness Program aimed at achieving health, happiness, and harmony in all areas of life, promoting holistic well-being and balance.

Life lessons indeed offer a powerful roadmap for personal growth and fulfillment. Each lesson guides us through experiences, shaping our perspectives and expectations. Let's delve deeper into how these lessons impact us:

Learning :

A Path to Personal and Spiritual Growth

1. **Continuous Growth:** Learning doesn't stop with school; it's a lifelong journey. This continuous learning helps us adapt, grow, and improve over time.

2. **Self-Awareness:** Learning helps us understand who we are. By gaining insights into our emotions, strengths, and weaknesses, we become more aware of how to improve ourselves

3. **Spiritual Development:** Learning isn't just about gaining knowledge. It also includes spiritual growth through practices like meditation. These practices help us connect with our inner selves, find inner peace, and understand life's deeper meanings.

4. **Transforming through Learning:** Continuous learning transforms us. By unlearning negative habits and embracing positive changes, we improve both our own lives and the lives of those around us.

5. **Learning from Others:** We can learn a lot by observing and listening to others. Mentors, family members, and even peers can provide insights and lessons that enrich our personal and professional lives.

6. **Self-Learning:** In today's world, the ability to teach yourself new skills is vital. Whether through online resources, books etc.

7. **Critical Thinking:** Learning develops critical thinking skills. By questioning, analyzing, and understanding different perspectives, we make more informed decisions

Earning :

A Holistic Approach to Wealth and Happiness

1. **1. Balancing Work and Life:** True earning means balancing our jobs with personal happiness. It's essential to take care of our health and relationships too.

2. **Spiritual Earning:** Earning isn't just about money. Engaging in work that aligns with our values and contributes to the community brings spiritual wealth, helping us live a more purposeful life.

3. **Building Goodwill:** Goodwill is earned through kindness, honesty, and positive actions. While it can't be measured in money, it strengthens relationships and adds a deeper richness to life that goes beyond material wealth.

4. **Giving Back to Community:** True earning also involves giving back—through charity, community service, or mentorship. When we help others, we make the world a better place, improving their lives and ours too.

5. **Earning Knowledge:** Spending time every day on self-improvement and personal growth is really important. It helps you see challenges from a new perspective. With knowledge, you can

make better choices and face problems with confidence. Reading books is one of the best ways for self-improvement and self-growth.

6. **Emotional wealth:** Many of us focus on making money but overlook emotional wealth, which is equally important. A life rich in love, gratitude and meaningful relationships truly matters.

7. **Earning Respect:** Respect both for yourself and from others, needs to be earned through being honest, kind, and reliable. It's a type of wealth that builds character and strengthens relationships.

Expectation :

The Key to Managing Balance and Motivation

1. **Setting Realistic Goals:** Expectations guide us toward our goals. By setting realistic and meaningful expectations, we can achieve personal growth and professional success without unnecessary stress.

2. **Managing Disappointment:** Unrealistic expectations can gives some time gives disappointment. Learning to manage expectations will helps us handle setbacks and maintain emotional balance.

3. **Finding Inner Peace**: When we align our expectations with our values and focus on the journey, we can find inner peace. This helps reduce stress and lets us enjoy life more.

4. **Healthy Expectations in Relationships**: Setting realistic expectations in relationships with family, friends, or coworkers helps create better connections. Good communication and understanding can prevent conflicts and build harmony.

5. **Expectations and Self-Improvement:** Having goals for yourself, like wanting to improve and reach personal milestones, can inspire growth. But it's important to be kind to yourself and be patient as you work toward these goals.

6. **Expectation vs. Reality Check:** It's important to regularly check if our expectations match reality. Adjusting them to what's possible helps us stay balanced and reduces stress.

7. **Expectations and Gratitude**: Focusing on what we have instead of what we lack helps us set realistic expectations and feel more content. Practicing gratitude brings a sense of humbleness and makes us appreciate life more.

These key points for learning, earning and expectations highlight how a balanced approach can lead to a fulfilling life. When we focus on personal growth, holistic wealth, and managing expectations, we cultivate a life filled with meaning, happiness, and well-being.

|| ॐ ||

Himani Verma

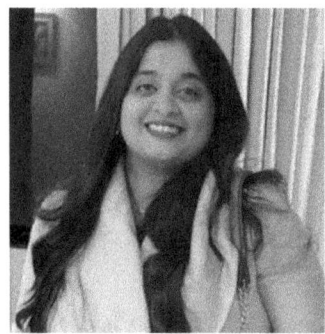

Author's Name	:	Himani Verma
Qualification	:	M.Sc. (Chemistry), B.Ed.
Current Profession	:	Educator
Age	:	29 years
E-mail ID	:	**himani221294@gmail.com**
City/ Country	:	**Punjab, India**

Himani Verma is an accomplished educator with a Master Degree in Chemistry. With a robust teaching career spanning over four years, she currently imparts her knowledge and passion for the subject at Quest International School. Known for her dedication and innovative teaching methods,

Himani has become a respected figure in the academic community, inspiring her students to excel in Chemistry and beyond.

LEE, The Learning, Earning and Expectation are some inter-related facts of life that shape any individual's holistic development. Learning is a lifelong journey which consist not only formal education, but also the values, ethics, set of morals that shape us to be a better person. On the contrary, Earning is an impalpable outcome of learning. Earning not only arises from the materialistic assets but also the love, respect, harmony in relationships, serenity in behavior are phenomenal facets of learning.

Learning :

1. **Unconditional Love:** The bedrock of life, what we call is love. Work-Life balance is imperative: Whether it's balancing personal ambitions with shared dreams or balancing work with family life, this learning will be cherished forever.

2. **Adaptability:** Teaching has taught me that patience is a key virtue, not just in the classroom but in all walks of life, those who are able to adapt to varied circumstances are true fighters.

3. **Health is the fortune:** Maintaining a good health is the par-important thing one can have in life.

4. **The universe returns what you put it into:** Our karmic account is what makes our past, present and future.
5. **Wisdom:** Life is constantly evolving, and wisdom involves recognizing that change is inevitable.
6. **Empathy:** Empathy teaches us to be more considerate towards the feelings of people surrounding us.
7. **Family above all:** This learning is the mirror which reflects that life is merely not composed of materialistic wealth but with the persons in it whom we call our home.

Earning :

1. **Inner Peace and Contentment:** Traversing the journey, one gains the invaluable sense of contentment and inner peace, realizing that true wealth lies in the experiences, love, and lessons you've accumulated rather than in material possessions.
2. **Family's Love:** The purest form of love lies here, the sense of belongingness and acceptance.
3. **Embracing your roots:** The culture and the creed from where we come should be deeply instilled in us.
4. **Respect:** One of the most important earning in one's life is earning is respect which allow an individual to accept somebody for who they are.
5. **Character and Integrity:** Building a reputation based on honesty, integrity, and ethical behavior is a significant intangible asset.
6. **Spiritual Fulfillment:** Spiritual growth and fulfillment, whether through religious beliefs, meditation, or personal philosophies, provide a deeper sense of purpose and peace.
7. **Attracting Goodwill's:** Counting your blessings showered by your loved one is the biggest earning that we can acquire in life.

Expectation :

Peace and Contentment: Living a a peaceful life with self respect and emancipation is the ultimate goal.

Learning should go on: Life never stops teaching so never stop developing yourself and your skills.

Growth : Continuously developing skills, knowledge, and character.

Security: Attaining financial stability and safety.

Exploratory living: Experiencing new and exciting opportunities.

Work-Life balance: Leading a life with a harmonious balance of work and professional life.

Legacy: Leaving positive imprints on others and world

|| ॐ ||

Isha Singh

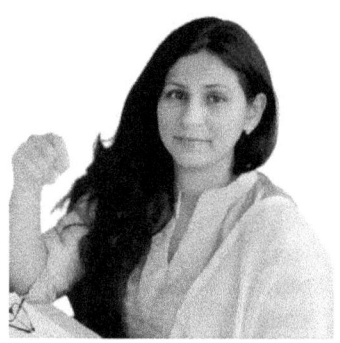

Author's Name	:	Isha Singh
Qualification	:	Pursuing MA Psychology, PG Diploma in Mass Communication
Current Profession	:	Graphologist, Drawing & Doodle Analyst, DOB Analyst, Parenting Coach and NLP Practitioner
Age	:	42 years
E-mail ID	:	**ishhasingh05@gmail.com**
City/ Country	:	**Gurugram, Haryana**

Isha Singh is a multidisciplinary expert in human behavior and development. With a Postgraduate Degree in Mass Communication and ongoing studies in Psychology, she has combined her knowledge with certifications in Graphology, DOB analysis, and NLP practice. As the founder of **Selfwrite Institute of Holistic Development**, Isha has spent over three years helping individuals understand themselves better through handwriting analysis, signature analysis and drawing analysis. Her expertise extends to parenting coaching, empowering parents to foster strong bonds with their children. Isha is dedicated to using her expertise to nurture the next generation's growth and well-being."

Throughout my life, learning has been the foundation of growth, shaping my values and perspectives. Earning has provided not only financial stability but also the freedom to pursue my passions. For me, these earnings are not measured by material wealth or external success, but by the richness of my heart, mind, and spirit, and the discovery of the best version of myself. My evolving expectations have guided me towards a life of purpose, where successes and setbacks are embraced with equal grace. Living fully means cherishing each moment, nurturing relationships, and striving for personal and spiritual growth in every aspect of life. Remember, life is unpredictable and expectations can vary; be open-minded, flexible and kind to yourself and others.

Learning:

1. **Embrace Imperfection:** Embrace your flaws and those of others, nobody is perfect, and that's okay.
2. **Practice Self-Love:** Love yourself first, and you'll find it easier to love others.
3. **Forgive and Let Go:** Holding grudges weighs you down, forgive and move on.
4. **Be Present:** Life happens in the present moment so focus on now, not yesterday or tomorrow.
5. **Take Responsibility:** Own your actions and decisions as blaming others won't help you grow.
6. **Embrace Challenges:** Embrace Life's challenges as an opportunity for your personal growth.
7. **Practice Gratitude:** Gratitude opens doors to happiness so focus on what you have, not what you lack.

Earning :

1. **Wisdom:** Earn wisdom by learning from experiences and applying it to make better decisions.
2. **Respect:** Earn respect from others by being kind, empathetic and genuine.
3. **Love:** Earn love by nurturing relationships and showing compassion and care.
4. **Personal Growth:** Earn a sense of personal growth by pushing beyond your comfort zone and developing new skills.
5. **Inner Peace:** Earn inner peace by cultivating mindfulness, gratitude, and self-awareness.
6. **Memories:** Earn cherished memories by creating experiences and sharing moments with loved ones.
7. **Legacy:** Earn a lasting legacy by making a positive impact on the world and leaving a footprint that inspires others.

Expectation:

1. **Change:** Embrace change, it's inevitable and can bring new opportunities.
2. **Consistency**: Expect consistency in effort, not outcome. Stay committed to your values and goals, even when faced with obstacles or uncertainties.
3. **Setbacks:** Setbacks are part and parcel of life face it with resilience and perseverance.
4. **Growth:** Personal growth is a lifelong journey; expect to learn and evolve.
5. **Relationship matters:** Nurture relationships, as they bring joy, support, and happiness.
6. **Surprises:** Life is full of surprises accept it as either good or bad.
7. **Adaptability:** Stay adaptable and open to new experiences, perspectives, and learning opportunities.

|| ॐ ||

Jiggna B Bhatt

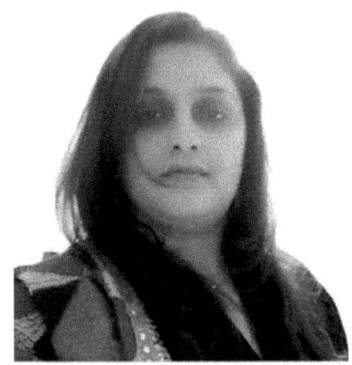

Author's Name	:	Jiggna B Bhatt
Qualification	:	Graduate in Commerce & Diploma in Software Engineering
Current Profession	:	Entrepreneur Deals in Rudraksh, Crystal and other Products used in Occult Science – Astrology, Numerology and Vastu etc.
Age	:	41 Years
E-mail ID	:	**jiggnabhattzee@gmail.com**
City/ Country	:	**Dubai, UAE**

Jiggna B Bhatt is a renowed Rudraksh and Vastu Specialist. She also specialises in Crystal remedies and Numerology. Jigggna B Bhatt has done her Graduation from Mumbai University and had been working as Banking Professional in UAE for almost 10 years. Presently she is a professional Occult Practitioner.

Being associated with many renowned senior Numerologists and Occult Practitioners like **Abhishaik Chitraans** of **M/s Ankakshr Miracless,** she has learnt many new methodologies in Numerology and has tried and helped many individual/ business houses in India and UAE as well.

Being a vastu and rudraksh specialist more than 1000+ clients have been advised and improved their lives and houses/ families across UAE, UK and India. Occult and Rudraksh products prescribed by her are really awesome.

In the journey of life, the *Seven LEE* – Learnings, Earnings and Expectations – serve as pillars of personal growth and fulfillment. Learnings ground us, providing insights at every phase, from wonder in childhood to acceptance in later years. Earnings represent the intangible wealth we gather, like wisdom, resilience and joy, which enrich our spirit. Expectations drive our aspirations, pushing us to discover, achieve and leave a legacy. Together, these elements create a life of depth and purpose, turning everyday experiences into a unique story. Embracing the Seven LEE helps us live meaningfully, leaving a lasting impact.

Learning :

1. **Wonder** – Childhood teaches us to be endlessly curious and open to the world's magic.
2. **Courage** – Adolescence instills bravery, as we face the unknown and begin to shape our identities.
3. **Purpose** – Young adulthood drives us to find meaning and set goals, defining our path.
4. **Balance** – In adulthood, we learn to juggle responsibilities, finding harmony between personal and professional lives.
5. **Gratitude** – Midlife brings the wisdom of appreciation for what we have and who we are.
6. **Legacy** – In later years, we focus on what we leave behind, nurturing relationships and passing down wisdom.
7. **Acceptance** – In our final phase, we find peace in letting go, embracing the journey as it was meant to be.

Earning :

1. **Wisdom** – From experiences, both good and challenging, we gain knowledge that shapes our perspectives.
2. **Resilience** – Life's trials build our inner strength, teaching us to rise each time we fall.
3. **Connections** – Relationships add joy and meaning, teaching us the value of empathy and support.
4. **Joy** – The simple moments remind us to celebrate, making life lighter and more fulfilling.
5. **Contentment** – Accepting ourselves and our lives as they are brings peace, reducing the need for constant striving.
6. **Gratitude** – Recognizing our blessings, big or small, helps us appreciate the journey and stay grounded.
7. **Legacy** – Through actions and kindness, we create a positive impact that lives on, enriching future generations.

Expectation :

1. **Discovery** – In childhood, we expect to explore, learn, and understand the world around us.
2. **Identity** – In adolescence, we seek self-understanding, hoping to discover who we truly are.

3. **Achievement** – Young adulthood fills us with ambition; we expect to reach goals and make a name for ourselves.

4. **Belonging** – In adulthood, we crave connection and acceptance, seeking a place where we truly fit in.

5. **Fulfilment** – Midlife brings the desire to feel complete, to live in alignment with our values and purpose.

6. **Impact** – In later years, we hope to contribute positively, leaving behind a legacy that reflects our life's values.

7. **Peace** – Nearing the end, we long for tranquillity, expecting to find closure, contentment, and acceptance.

॥ ॐ ॥

Kala Malpani

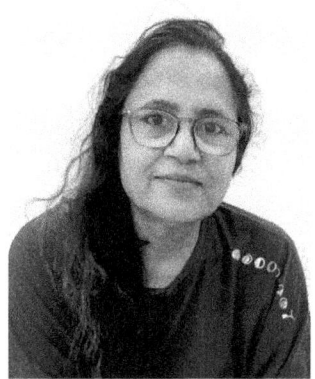

Author's Name	:	Kala Malpani
Qualification	:	HS, Certified Graphologist, Numerologist, Grapho-therapist, Logo Analyst & Designer
Current Profession	:	Graphologist, Numerologist
Age	:	64 years (45 years of Married Life)
E-mail ID	:	**malpanikala1@gmail.com**
City/ Country	:	**Mumbai, India**

Kala Malpani is a professional Graphologist, have been pursuing Graphology since 2011. She has a vast experience of teaching online and counselling in person. She has conducted more than 50 sessions in various collages n schools of cities like Mumbai-Bangalore, including medical institutions also. She has experience of doing corporate events in India as well as abroad. Her expertise is Grapho-therapy & Handwriting development. She is a numerologist and Logo analyst n designer too.

Besides all these she is socially active in her community organisations and have taken various posts there. She has performed responsibilities of different posts in organisations like Lions club also. Before coming in the field of Graphology, she was a renowned dress designer. There also she had a wide experience of 20 years. She was running a boutique successfully.

On top of all the above-mentioned fields, she is a homemaker, the area close to her heart.

Kala Malpani's rich background and diverse expertise make her a multifaceted professional, dedicated to her career, community and family.

'Seven LEE of Life', refers to ***Learning, Earning*** and ***Expectation***; each of these categories contains seven aspects of life. These aspects represent a comprehensive framework for living a purposeful, engaging and meaningful life.

When I look back into my life, it seems, I've experienced sorrow and joy with a deep sense of synchronicity in my life, where everything seems to unfold at just the right moment to embrace both, the highs and lows.

This perspective shows a remarkable ability to understand that each has its place and purpose. This understanding has shaped the way I approach new challenges and opportunities. Whenever I faced challenges, I came out stronger. And relished joyful experiences with more zest. My faith on divine plan have become stronger.

And these experiences gave the great learnings of life, gave insight on my self-awareness: am able to reflect on my life and identify patterns and navigate life in future

Here are the main points of each LEEs :

Learning :

1. I strongly believe in the theory of thoughts, that our thoughts significantly impact our lives, influencing our health, wealth and relationships.

2. I have learnt that positive thinking and affirmations are just the first step, true transformation requires aligning my actions, habits and mindset to match my goals and aspirations.

3. Through my struggles with ailments, I discovered the power of my thoughts and learned a valuable lesson that every specific body organ is linked with each specific thought and changing thought can revert physical condition also.

4. Through my mistakes, I've gained valuable insights on how to manifest my desires and avoid common pitfalls where others often astray. For example, when I become desperate, the manifestation process slows down. However, when I put a thought into the universe and let it fly like a butterfly, it returns to me naturally and effortlessly. This approach taught me the importance of patience and trust in the process, allowing things to unfold in their own time without forcing outcomes.

5. I believe that just like every coin has two sides, every situation has its pros n cons. It's up to us to choose which side we focus on and how we approach it.

6. Give your 100% wherever you are and whatever you do. Perform with your full capacity, passion and dedication. For example, when you're working on a project, immerse yourself fully in it, paying attention to every detail, will bring excellence in your work. If you're spending time with family, be fully present and engage with them wholeheartedly, will create meaningful connections. Whether professional task or personal, my approach with this mindset not only leaded to better outcomes but also brought fulfilment.

7. Our emotions are fluid and change over time, even towards the same person, we often go through phases where feelings of love, affection, or even resentment can fluctuate. These

changes can be influenced by various factors such as circumstances, misunderstandings, personal growth, or external stressors.

Earning :

1. The greatest wealth I've accumulated in my life is the love and connection I share with my family and friends.
2. I have a rich and reflective life journey, every experience, exhilarating or excruciating, both has offered priceless insights and contributed to my growth in life.
3. Being regarded with respect and esteem by those I value, is also a significant accomplishment of my life.
4. Establishing a strong social presence and being recognized with my community is another accomplishment, I am proud of.
5. My childlike nature is a treasure, it allows me to approach life with excitement, curiosity and a sense of adventure.
6. Maintaining my health and looks is not just about external appearance, but also about feeling strong, confident and vibrant from the inside out.
7. To be introduced to Graphology, came in life as serendipitous blessing and turned around my life 180 degrees.

Expectation :

1. I wish to have good health, both, physical as well as mental till my last breath.
2. I wish for my loved ones to live a life with happiness, contentment and fulfilment.
3. May my dedication towards my nation and Hinduism yield fruitful and positive outcome.
4. May my efforts and achievements be etched in the memories of those I've touched, creating a timeless legacy that continues to uplift and motivate others long after I'm gone."
5. May I rise to elevated states of spiritual realms, deepening my connections with Divine and cultivating inner peace, wisdom and compassion.
6. Since I have experienced the benefits of living in present moment, expect to be always in that mindset
7. May my life story conclude with fulfilled and serene ending.

Kalpana Priyadarshi

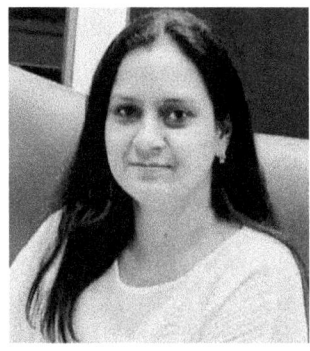

Author's Name	:	Kalpana Priyadarshi
Qualification	:	B.Sc., B.Ed., M.Sc.
Current Profession	:	Teacher
Age	:	42
E-mail ID	:	…
City/ Country	:	**Bengaluru, India**

Kalpana Priyadarshi is a teacher and a writer. She has done her Master Degree in Biotechnology. She has graduated in life sciences.

She is also graduated in Education in physical science and life science.

Kalpana Priyadarshi, loves to write about society, life and feelings. Her writings have got special emphasis on the lives, conditions and feelings of females and the effects of society on their lives.

Kalpana has the below LEEs of life :

Learning :

1. **You are important:** You are the most important in this world, know this truth. Take care of your physical and mental health.

2. **You are what you speak:** Your definition is shaped from the content which comes out of your mouth.

3. **Education is never complete:** Seek knowledge and continue learning. Keep on learning a new thing, irrespective of age and situation.

4. **Rule yourself:** Rule your mind or it will rule you.
5. **Forgive:** Forgiveness benefits two people, the giver and the receiver.
6. **Have a porpose:** Life is incomplete without a purpose, make sure to have a purpose always.
7. **Live in positivity:** Surround yourself with positive people.

Earning :

1. **Health:** focus on earning health, it's a great treasure.
2. **Family and Friends:** focus on counting family and friends in life.
3. **Values:** values which we attain through the lifetime are the real bank balance.
4. **Experiences and Memories:** the experiences we learn in our life through the ups and downs and memories we create good or bad, are the real earnings.
5. **Wisdom and Knowledge:** the wisdom and knowledge attained throughout the life.
6. **Self-love:** loving oneself is the greatest earnings if we could attain.
7. **Respect from people:** getting respect from people in life is a good earning.

Expectation :

1. **Discipline:** expect discipline from yourself.
2. **Imperfections:** imperfections can be there in relationships and situations.
3. **Peace:** expect peace at your heart.
4. **Self-expectations:** Always expect maximum from yourself.
5. **Smile:** Have a smile on your lips no matter what.
6. **Gratefulness:** My heart becomes grateful for everything.
7. **Forgiveness:** I can forgive everyone and everything.

|| ॐ ||

Kanan Jolly

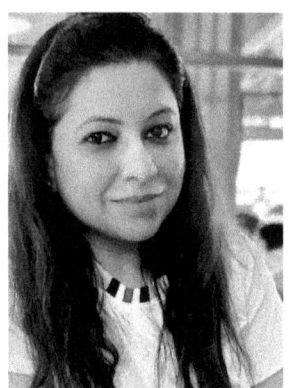

Author's Name	:	Kanan Jolly
Qualification	:	Graduate in Computer Science, Software Engineer
Current Profession	:	Working with MNC as Assistant Vice President
Age	:	43 Years
E-mail ID	:	**lifecoachkananj@gmail.com**
City/ Country	:	**Mumbai, India**

Kanan Jolly is a working professional and a happy single parent to a 13-year-old son. She is also playing a role of Certified Life Coach, Numerologist, Tarot and Angel Card Reader, also practicing NLP & Access Consciousness. She is a Motivational Speaker & Author. She is passionate about empowering Women to unlock their potential and have meaningful results in their lives. She is a Single Parent to a loving Son. She is a manifestor of the beautiful life, she is living.

It's always our choice to learn the lesson and evolve or keep repeating the same mistakes. Number-7 is the number of wisdom and research, this number also depicts just like the 7 colours of the rainbow how colourful our life can be if we keep evolving and learning. I am in deep Gratitude for all the learnings I have gained in this lifetime, each experience good or bad has contributed to my life. All the learnings from my childhood to my teens, from school to college to my career each situation has taught me a lesson. While growing up I was told I should value others more than myself and in the process of keeping everyone happy I stopped valuing myself, however, when I started focusing on myself that is when I learnt the '*Seven LEE of life*', which I shared below for those who are willing to transform their life. I wish all the readers all the best and may you learn & implement the *Seven LEE of life* shared in this book.

Learning :

1) Live in Gratitude and focus on possibilities, so that you can create more opportunities.
2) Always be present, by being aligned with your mind, heart, and body for better experiences in life.
3) People you meet in life come with an agenda, a purpose either to teach you or to learn from you.
4) Spend your money wisely and save more, with the intention that you will use it for your Happy Days.
5) Don't take everything so personally as nobody thinks about you as much as you do.
6) Listen to your body and be present to it, by doing this you can have a better healthier body & life.
7) Save your energy by speaking only when it's required as control over your tongue can have control over your future.

Earning :

1. Good deeds, good **Karma** and good actions are earnings of life, our value system always keeps us on the right path.
2. **Blessings** are just like a boomerang the more you give the more you get so keep blessing others to receive more.
3. As a being the unconditional **Love** that we receive from our family and friends is a true earning.
4. As a soul, our **Wisdome & Awareness** help us to achieve the learnings we have chosen to experience before coming to this planet.
5. All the **Memories** that we create & live with our family and friends are our lifetime experiences and earnings.
6. We all have experienced **Miracles** in our lives, it says the Universe is always with us and that's an earning for me.
7. A healthy **Mind & Body**, inner peace, mental well-being is a real blessing.

Expectation :

1) **Spirituality:** To live life as a Spiritual being, to learn, experience, grow and evolve in this lifetime.
2) **Finances:** To live life with financial freedom, to freely contribute to society.
3) **Memories:** To create and live beautiful moments with my Family which will be my lifetime memories.
4) **Wisdom:** To live my life as a lifelong learner so that learnings & wisdom can keep me on the right path.
5) **Growth:** To grow in my professional life and career, growth in whatever I choose to do.

6) **Desire:** All my materialistic desires to come true in this lifetime.

7) **Travel:** To travel around the world, to learn about different cultures and traditions.

Gratitude!

॥ ॐ ॥

Kanchan Lakhwani

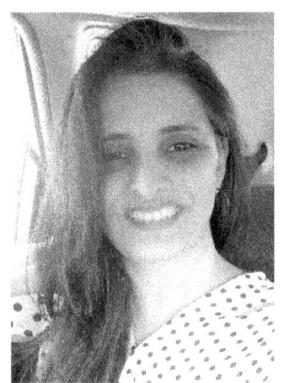

Author's Name	:	Kanchan Lakhwani
Qualification	:	B.A. in English (Lang. & Lit.)
Current Profession	:	Educationist (Student Tutor)
Age	:	44 years
E-mail ID	:	**harrshitagangwaanii@gmail.com**
City/ Country	:	**Mumbai, India**

Kanchan Lakhwani has completed her Bachelor's in English Language and Literature from Mumbai University. She is an Educationist and an Entrepreneur. She has been providing tuition services (for individual students and group) to IGCSE, ICSE and CBSE wards for more than two decades now. She strongly feels that being around children has kept her grounded and sane; giving her all the more reason to continue with the profession that she is in. She also runs her small business of healthy roasted seeds like watermelon, muskmelon and hemp etc. – as recommended to patients by the doctor – She delivers on a pre-order basis. Her major clientele comprises corporates, who order healthy hampers during festivities, to give to their employees.

Kanchan has won 'Most Beautiful Hair' title, in the prestigious 'Mrs Maharashtra Iconic Diva 2020 – supporting Fight Against Domestic Violence' pageant, held in January 2020. Women across many walks of life came together to express their support to women who silently go through domestic violence inside the four walls of their cocoon.

As there exist millions of people on this earth, there also exist an equal number of different mindsets. Its mind blowing howone particular topic can have such varied perspectives. Anthologies are a brilliant way to access these perspectives and a new viewpoint on subjects that we are conditioned to look at, in a particular way. They serve students and layman alike; to view the subject in a different light. An anthologist has a purpose in mind and openly invites authors from various backgrounds to submit their works; the more the authors, the more the flavour in the book. It's as much fun for the anthologist to compile the collections as it is for the readers to witness a culmination of one idea from innumerable variations.

Learning :

1. Work - continue working and don't be attached to the result

2. Flexiblitlity - be flexible with things that matter

3. Let live - live and let live, we are all here to perform our part

4. Be honest - you will never have to remember things if you are honest.

5. Work smart - with so much evolution happening, utilise the tools available and work smart

6. Responsibility - taking up responsibilities helps you grow as an individual

7. Care - caring for your close ones gives a different high and satisfaction

Earning :

1. Respect - respect comes when we put ourselves in the other person's shoe

2. Love - love your family and friends unconditionally

3. Self confidence - with the support of family and friends even negative self confidence can be restored

4. Loyalty - stay loyal for your own peace of mind

5. Education - continue your education till your last breath and keep growing each day

6. Leadership - lead good causes to feel a sense of contentment

7. Personality - be in the company of positive people and individuals who are more experienced, to develop a overall personality

Expectation :

1. Love - An expression of love from family and friends would work wonders

2. Respect - A respectful relationship where everyone is equally heard

3. Communication - an open communication can work wonders for life

4. Family - A complete satisfied family where responsibilities are shared with openness

5. Money - More money so investments and expenses can be taken care of easily and a comfortable life is lived

6. Bigger home - where the entire family and extended family can live happily

7. Religious - many religious classes are attended for the growth of the soul.

|| ॐ ||

Kavitha Bhutada

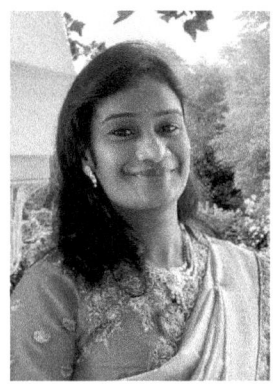

Author's Name	:	Kavitha Bhutada
Qualification	:	M.B.A., B.Ed.
Current Profession	:	Teacher
Age	:	38 years
E-mail ID	:	**sonikavitha111.ks@gmail.com**
City/ Country	:	**Mysore, India**

Kavitha Bhutada is an M.B.A. graduate and holds a B.Ed. degree pursued when she wanted to transform her passion of teaching into reality, currently working as a dedicated teacher. Alongside her professional career, she is a passionate artist with a talent for painting and a flair of creativity. She excels at various forms of craft, bringing her ideas to life with intricate designs and thoughtful details.

Kavitha is an accomplished homemaker. She is capable to balance her career and personal life, while nurturing her role as mother of two. As a mother, she is deeply committed in fostering her children's growth, providing them with love, guidance and the values needed to navigate life. She believes in nurturing their creativity and independence, always striving to be a source of encouragement and strength. Through her experiences, she brings a unique perspective on the journey of marriage, exploring the joys and challenges with authenticity and insight

'Seven lee of Life' is a mantra for achieving the goals. These 7 LEEs will inspire, motivate and help you to work towards the betterment of life."Learning, Earning and expectation" are the three LEE and I have written the 7 points to unravel it :

Learning:

1. **Excitement** - to learn something new
2. **Resilience** - Developing Resilience to bounce back even after failures
3. **Adaptability** - Adapting new changes and updating ourselves
4. **Collaboration** - Collaborating with intellectual people
5. **Analysis** - Critical understanding of experiences and knowledge.
6. **Goal setting** - Setting goals to guide your learning journey and achieve them
7. **Never ending process** - Learning is a continuous process and work towards personal and professional growth.

Earning:

1. **Education** - Invest in learning to expand skills and knowledge
2. **Work ethic** - Hard work and dedication often leads to financial success
3. **Networking** - Building strong professional relationships can open new earning opportunities
4. **Innovation** - Creative thinking and innovation can lead to profitable ventures.
5. **Financial Management** - Wise management of earnings is crucial for long term wealth
6. **Adaptability** - Being adaptable allows you to seize new earnings
7. **Persistence** - Staying persistent, even in the face of setbacks, is the key.

Expectation:

1. **Real** - ground your expectations in reality to avoid disappointments
2. **Flexibility** - stay open to change and adapt if needed.
3. **Patience** - understand that good things often take time to manifest
4. **Gratitude** - Appreciate what you have while striving for more.
5. **Communication** - Clearly express your expectations to others to avoid misunderstanding.
6. **Mindfulness** - Stay present and avoid letting future expectations overshadow the current moment.
7. **Resilience** - Bounce back from the failures and view them as learning opportunities.

|| ॐ ||

Keerthika

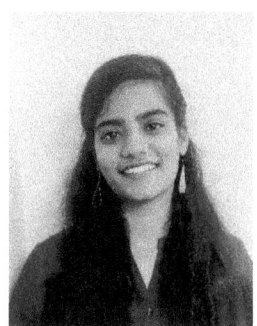

Author's Name	:	Keerthika
Qualification	:	B.E, (Bachelor of Electronics & Instrumentation Engg.)
Current Profession	:	Engineer
Age	:	26 years
E-mail ID	:	**keerthikab297@gmail.com**
City/ Country	:	**Bangalore, India**

Keerthika is the debut co-author of this book you are reading now and also a dedicated Engineer with a growing passion for writing. Alongside her budding literary career, she is deeply enthusiastic about cooking and is a nature lover who enjoys travelling.

She completed her Bachelors in Electronics and Instrumentation Engineering at Madras Institute of Technology Campus, Anna University and has been working for nearly five years as an Engineer in the Oil and Gas sector.

Rooted in a humble background, she constantly seeks opportunities that foster both professional and personal growth. She embraces new challenges with enthusiasm and is driven by a constant desire to explore and expand her horizons. Beyond her Engineering profession, she is dedicated to her culinary pursuits and writing, reflecting her diverse interests and talents.

This book is a testament to her passion for writing and she hereby shares her views on the title of the book as a co-author.

'Seven LEE of Life' is a profound phrase that encapsulates the essence of one's entire life. There is a saying that goes, "When you look back to your life, make sure it's worth watching." This concept not only echoes that sentiment but also encourages us to pause in this fast-paced world, to reflect on what we have done, and to consider what we aspire to become. As an anthology of insights from 108 authors, this book is sure to offer a multitude of perspectives on how to approach life moving forward.

Learning :

1. Being Honest to oneself in the first place
2. Staying Focused
3. Understanding between do's and don'ts
4. Control of mind and heart according to the situation
5. Disciplined way of life
6. Self satisfaction is important.No need to please anyone
7. Live for oneself but not for the society

Earning :

1. Good people for myself
2. Anger management
3. Decision making skills
4. Managing many things by proper planning
5. Self discipline
6. Respect
7. Love and care

Expectation :

1. Getting rid of laziness totally
2. Zero procrastination
3. Choosing healthier way of life over likings
4. Travel around the world more and learn
5. Not falling in the trap of emotions
6. To live the present moment everyday without worrying much about future
7. Reduce overthinking

|| ॐ ||

Kiran Yadav

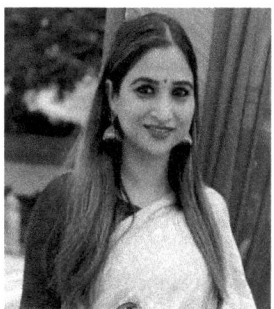

Author's Name	:	Kiran Yadav
Qualification	:	M.Com, M.B.A
Current Profession	:	Business woman
Age	:	36 years
E-mail ID	:	**kirany15487@gmail.com**
City/ Country	:	**Gurgaon, India**

Kiran Yadav is a Fantastic Educator. She has done her Master's Degrees in Commerce and Business Administration and holds a degree in Education. She has worked for more than 8 years as HR in reputed MNCs and the Hotel Industry. She has conducted many pieces of training for the fresher; later on, she was employed at various renowned International schools in Gurugram, India as a PRT Teacher.

She loves to enjoy nature strolls and listening to music.

She strongly believes if you love yourself, it's easy for you to spread love everywhere. It will help you to stay positive always.

Knock ! The manner in which you see life, significantly alters the manner in which you experience it, while my mother taught me to be self-reliant, my father taught me to be fearless, gained the art of selfless service from my better half, how to uninhibitedly giggle from my children, society taught me the respect that accompanies with popularity and business taught me to win even after losing.

"A genuine individual is one who battles with the circumstances and makes his life effective and works on the existence of himself as well as individuals connected with him."

Whenever I feel that I have lost, I recollect these 4 lines and I don't have a clue about the wellspring of solidarity that keeps me pushing ahead and makes me stand tall fearlessly.

It's something to that effect, I'm saying, "I'm not one of the people who lose in this life", proceed to thump on another person's entryway, here my triumph is sure.

Learning:

1. **Bow down:** I have learned to bow down for the happiness of my loved ones in life
2. **Patience:** be patient, patience helps you to make right decisions for a smoother life.
3. **Giver:** I have learned to give, there is no greater happiness than giving
4. **There is only one You, who can find yourself from the core of your heart**
5. Never please anyone for your happiness
6. Don't forget your roots from where you came from
7. Do not compromise on your dreams, be focused

Earning:

1. **Respect:** Respect is the basis of your life actions
2. **Humanity:** The humanity inside you connects you with the divine
3. **Stability:** there is no end to desires that's why stability is must.
4. **Gratification:** Mental satisfaction is more pleasurable then being successful in life.
5. I surround myself with right People.
6. Being fearless and Take risks.
7. **Resilience:** I have strategies for dealing with stress, adversity and trauma.

Expectation:

1. **Peace:** Achieving a peace that is a goal itself
2. **Liberty:** Liberty to express my own opinion
3. **Trust:** It's hard for me to Trust, so I want to learn to trust
4. **Growth:** Always want to move forward while working in life with unexpected Growth
5. **Triumph (a victory):** like Arjuna, I have my eyes set on my target and believe that I will achieve victory one day
6. **Support:** Always need support from my loved ones
7. **Renown:** A status that gives me recognition in my life

|| ॐ ||

Lalit Sharma

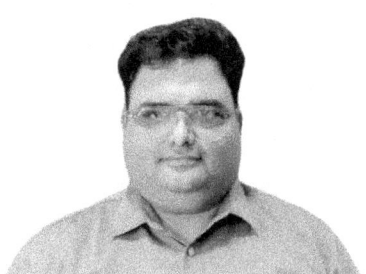

Author's Name	:	Lalit Sharma
Qualification	:	Under Graduate Certified Master Numerologist, Certified Vastu Advisor, Certified Palmist, Certified Astrologer, Certified Akashic Records Practitioner, Certified Meditation Practitioner, Psychic Healer
Current Profession	:	Occult Science Practitioner and Consultant
Age	:	48 years
E-mail ID	:	**anksatva@gmail.com**
City/ Country	:	**New Delhi, India**

Lalit Sharma is a distinguished occult practitioner with over three decades of experience in the fields of Numerology and Vastu Shastra. An internationally certified expert, Lalit has honed his skills through rigorous training at Bharatiya Vidya Bhawa, New Delhi and various prestigious institutes across India and Malaysia.

In 2015, he founded **Anksatva Academy**, a registered MSME and ISO Certified Institute dedicated to the study and practice of occult sciences. His academy offers a comprehensive curriculum that empowers students to explore and excel in their spiritual journeys.

Lalit is deeply committed to social causes and has actively participated in several initiatives aimed at environmental conservation and family welfare. He has volunteered with NGOs, contributing to projects like the CMS survey of the River Yamuna, as well as participating in movements such as Yamuna Satyagrah and Jal Sansad. Through his multifaceted expertise and community involvement, Lalit Sharma continues to inspire others on their spiritual paths while advocating for environmental and social change.

Life is an incredible journey, filled with experiences that shape our identities and destinies. The **'Seven LEE of Life'** illuminate the essential learnings, earnings and expectations we encounter along the way. The wisdom imparted by our parents and teachers lingers in our minds, guiding us through life's twists and turns.

Seven Universal Principles to be Learned :

1. Honesty is the best policy.
2. Treat others as you wish to be treated.
3. Good manners open doors.
4. Life doesn't always grant your wishes.
5. Success is born from hard work.
6. It's not always about you—share the stage.
7. Embrace responsibility with pride.

Learning :

In an ever-evolving world, the ability to learn continuously is paramount. Here are the core elements that define our growth:

1. **Empathy:** Cultivating a deep understanding of others' perspectives fosters genuine connections and compassion.
2. **Creative Problem Solving:** Embrace challenges as opportunities to think outside the box and overcome obstacles with innovation.
3. **Trust:** Built on the pillars of reliability and integrity, trust is the foundation of meaningful relationships. Nurture it carefully.
4. **Harnessing Anger:** Channel anger into positive action or creativity—it can be a powerful catalyst for change.
5. **Let Go of People-Pleasing:** While it's natural to seek validation, remember that you can't please everyone. Prioritize your own well-being.
6. **Embrace Failure:** Life teaches us, like a gardener tending to plants, to accept setbacks, learn from them, and bloom again.
7. **Calmness:** The human life has too much noices outside and insisde both, need to be calm by body & mind.

Earning :

1. **Trust:** Building trust takes time and consistency; treasure it when it's earned.
2. **Self-Love:** Recognize your inherent worth and invite others to see your brilliance.
3. **Respect:** To be respected, practice respect—it's a two-way street.
4. **Smile Through Tears:** Finding joy amid struggle is a remarkable strength.

5. **Daily Recognition:** Earn respect through small, sincere gestures that uplift others.
6. **True Satisfaction:** Remember, fulfillment comes from within, not from possessions.
7. **Friendship:** Cherish relationships grounded in unconditional love and support.

Expectation :

1. **Embrace Accountability:** Own your choices and their consequences.
2. **Take Charge:** Be proactive and responsible in all your commitments.
3. **Nurture Curiosity:** Approach life with an open mind and a thirst for knowledge.
4. **Focus on Impact:** Strive to create meaningful change in your endeavors.
5. **Listen Generously:** Practice active listening; it strengthens connections.
6. **Speak with Honesty:** Communicate directly and openly for deeper understanding.
7. **Empower Those Around You:** Lift others up, and you'll create a community of strength.

By embracing the **Seven LEE of Life**, we equip ourselves with essential tools for personal growth and fulfillment. Focusing on learning, earning, and setting realistic expectations paves the way for a rich, meaningful existence. Let these principles guide you as you navigate your unique journey!

|| ॐ ||

Leena Lalwani

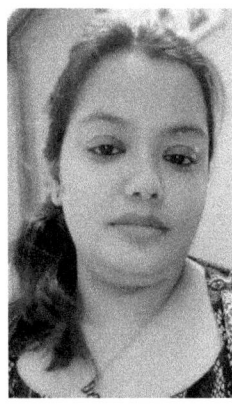

Author's Name	:	Leena Lalwani
Qualification	:	B.Com., Naturotherapist
Current Profession	:	Healer, Therapist, Numerologist
		Access Consciousness Bar Practitioner
Age	:	38 years
E-mail ID	:	**lalwanileena745@gmail.com**
City/ Country	:	**Mumbai, India**

Leena Lalwani is a Certified Therapist. She has done various therapies i.e Naturotherapy & Accutherapy. She is working in this profession morethan 10 years. She is also a Access Bars, Access Facelift & Body practitioner. She also practices as Numerologist and Tarot Card Reader. She has done Graduation in Commerce. She has changed lives of many people through her consultations and healing modelities.

She is also practices 8 modalities of healing and has successful results in Arthritis, Cancer, Depression, Parkinson, Dimentia, Asthma, Slip Disc, Cervical, Paralysis etc. She is also a Yoga Therapist and Yoga Trainer.

Leena Lalwani has the below LEEs of life :

Learning :

1. **Learning To Say No:** Learning to say no starts with understanding your limits and setting clear boundaries.

2. **Appreciate Your Journey:** Embrace your journey cause every steps shapes you.
3. **You Cant Please Everyone:** It maintain authenticity and build meaningful relationship with who appreciate you for who you are.
4. **Be Judgement-Free:** Being judgemental creates hurdles in your own success, So be judgement-free.
5. **Be The Best Version Of Yourself:** Be the best version of yourself by embracing your strength and continuously improving.
6. **Trust Your Gut Feelings:** Cause, Your gut often guides you towards the right decisions.
7. **Surrender To God:** It will unfold according to a higher plan by surrendering to God. We can feel and see the magic of our life.

Earning :

1. **My Intuition:** My intuitions to lead me in directions that align with my true self.
2. **Honesty:** I gained honest relationships with myself in my hard time.
3. **My Healing Power:** I have gained my healing power because of my pure intentions in my thoughts.
4. **Self-Dependent:** To be self-dependent one of my great earnings of my life.
5. **Trust Of My Clients:** I can proudly say that I earned trust of my clients.
6. **Good Communication:** While dealing with different kind of clients I became a good communicator.
7. **Knowledge & Wisdom:** In the past 7-8 years, I earned alot of wisdom about Occult Science profession.

Expectation :

1. **To Be A Good Social Activist:** I desire to be a good social activist and contribute to society.
2. **To Achieve My Dream House:** I desire to achieve my dream house and dream office in the upcoming future.
3. **To Become The Best Healer:** I desire to be the best healer and serve the best to my clients.
4. **NGO Founder:** I desire to run an NGO as an organiser and serve to society.
5. **To Achieve Success:** I desire to be a successful business woman.
6. **Entrepreneur:** I desire to be the best Entrepreneur of society.
7. **To Be The Best Consultant:** I desire to be the best consultant to my clients.

"Be the best version of yourself."

Lipiie Banerjjee

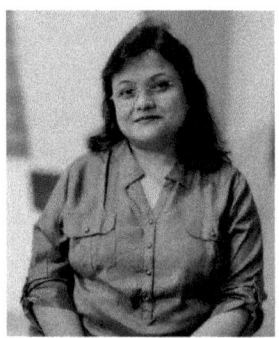

Author's Name	:	Lipiie Banerjjee
Qualification	:	B.Com., PGDBA
Current Profession	:	Consultant, Coach & Author
Age	:	54 years
E-mail ID	:	**banerjeelipi121@gmail.com**
City/ Country	:	**Mumbai, India**

Introducing a multifaceted and internationally renowned expert, **Lipiie Banerjjee** is an accomplished author whose works inspire and educate a global audience. As an NLP Trainer, she empowers individuals to unlock their potential through the power of language and mind. A Reiki Master, she provides healing and energy balancing, helping people achieve physical and emotional well-being. Her profound knowledge in Numerology and Astrology allows her to offer deep insights into life's patterns and cosmic influences.

She holds the prestigious titles of Gita Graduate and Advanced Vedantin reflecting her deep understanding of ancient spiritual wisdom and practices. Her journey from a successful corporate career to a dedicated spiritual catalyst is a testament to her commitment to personal growth and helping others. She combines her extensive expertise in various disciplines to guide individuals on their paths to self-discovery and transformation, making her a beacon of hope and change in the spiritual and personal development realms.

Lipiie says about the **LEE**s of Life :

Learnings: Life is a continuous journey of growth. Each experience, whether good or bad, adds to our understanding of the world and ourselves. Embracing these lessons with an open mind allows us to evolve, adapt, and ultimately live more fulfilling lives.

Earnings: Beyond material wealth, life offers intangible rewards like wisdom, love, and respect. These are the true treasures that define a successful life, enriching our existence in ways money cannot.

Expectations: While it's natural to have expectations, they can be a double-edged sword. Setting realistic expectations while remaining flexible can lead to contentment, while rigid expectations often lead to disappointment. Balancing aspirations with acceptance of life's unpredictability is the key to finding peace and satisfaction.

Learning :

1. **Embrace Change**: Change is inevitable and often leads to personal growth. Adaptability is crucial.
2. **Value Relationships**: Strong connections with others brings fulfillment and support during tough times.
3. **Practice Gratitude**: Recognizing the good in life fostered positivity and resilience.
4. **Pursue Passion**: Following what I love brings joy and purpose.
5. **Learn from Failure**: Mistakes are opportunities for growth, not just setbacks.
6. **Patience is Power**: Life often requires patience, as things unfold in their own time. Patience lead to deeper understanding and lasting success.
7. **Self-Compassion and Self-Love is Must**: Being kind to myself, especially during failures or hardships, is crucial for mental and emotional well-being. Self-compassion helps build resilience.

Earning :

1. **Emotional Earnings**: The deep satisfaction, joy, and fulfillment that comes from meaningful relationships, self-love, and inner peace.
2. **Intellectual Earnings**: The knowledge, wisdom, and skills I acquired through learning, curiosity, and experience.
3. **Spiritual Earnings**: The sense of purpose, connection, and inner harmony that I gained from spiritual practices, self-reflection, and understanding my place in the universe.
4. **Wisdom**: The deep understanding and insights gained from my life's challenges and lessons.
5. **Love**: The emotional connection and bonds formed with others, which brings fulfillment and support.
6. **Respect**: Earned through integrity, kindness, and actions that resonates with others.
7. **Legacy**: The impact and influence I will leave behind, shaping others' lives even after I am gone.

Expectation :

1. **Happiness, Love and Connection:**
2. **Success and Stability**
3. **Growth and Recognition**
4. **Recognition**
5. **Purpose**
6. **Fairness and Freedom**
7. **Adventure**

॥ ॐ ॥

Madhu Soni

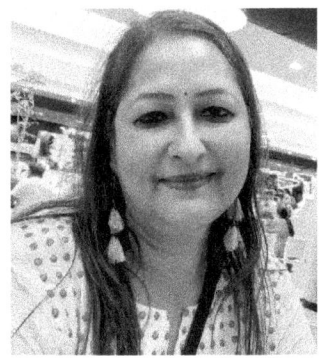

Author's Name	:	Madhu Soni
Qualification	:	Graduate
Current Profession	:	Graphologist, Grapho Therapist, Handwriting and Signature Consultant, Tarot Card Reader, Numerologist, Counselor, Coach and Mentor in moulding life.
Age	:	55 years
E-mail ID	:	**sonimadhusatish@gmail.com**
City/ Country	:	**Mumbai, India**

Madhu Soni is a multifaceted individual with a unique skill set that encompasses various fields such as graphology, drawing and signature analysis, doodle analysis, numerology, tarot card reading, handwriting analysis, grapho-therapy, and counseling for children. She possesses a deep understanding of human emotions and thought processes through which she provides valuable insights into analysing their personality sketch by underlying issues that may be affecting their personal and professional life.

Madhu Soni's unique blend of skills with her holistic approach reflects her unwavering commitment to empowering individuals of all ages to unlock their potential, overcome challenges and lead fulfilling lives guided by self-awareness and personal growth.

She has done various school projects about the awareness programme to improve handwriting for personality development. Apart from that she puts up stalls at exhibitions to encourage writing for self-improvement, focus and discipline.

She is the founder of **"miindgraphs" w**herein online/ offline consultations are done.

Madhu explains the **LEE** in terms of *'The Art and the Artist'* i.e.

Life is about learning and growing. We learn from our experiences and from others too. The experience comes with our actions towards the situations and the reactions we recieve and give. Both positive and negative virtues can be learnt easily depending on our ability and intelligence to handle a particular scenario. How smart sharp and quick we are the more things seems miniscule and manageable.

Earnings are essential financial stability and independence. It allows us to meet our basic needs and persue our goals and aspirations. However its a must to balance between work and personal life for smooth functioning. It also stands important because money, finance and tangible assets are overtaking every sphere and penetrating into the system like a monster. It is the thing, if I say so and attractive too. My opinion would be to strike a balance amongst the components as each has its own unique qualities.

Expectations play a significant role in shaping our perspective and determining our actions. It is crucial to set realistic expectations to avoid disappointment and frustration. Having a positive and grounded mindset can help us face life's challenges and setbacks in a more real, practical and honest way.

Learning :

1. My knowledge about the holistic approach towards life upgrading me.
2. Be focused and silent towards your goals.
3. Patience to deal with whatever may come
4. Listen to learn justifying two ears and one mouth given by God.
5. Speak your mind to be honest by virtue.
6. Make yourself a priority.
7. Love is the universal language most important to manage relationships.

Earnings :

1. People (Family & Friends, Clients & Students)
2. Money (Stability)
3. A super active mind which heals.
4. My experiences (Good & Bad)
5. My earned blessings of elders.
6. My gift of imparted teachings to the next generation.
7. My belief and value system.

Expectation :

1. Everyone is entitled to respect.
2. Happy vibes and love everywhere.
3. Financial security.
4. Mental security.
5. More opportunities to explore hidden talent inside me.
6. To get recognition worldwide.
7. To be instrumental in the work beneficial for my country.

At the end, Learning Earning and managing Expectation are essential for a meaningful and enriching life. It makes us content peaceful and happy to enjoy the moment, which comes our way.

|| ॐ ||

Manissha Shah

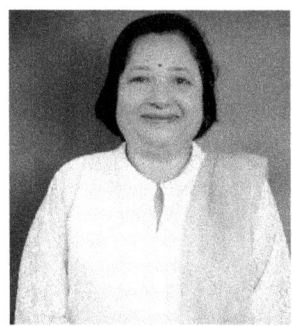

Author's Name	:	Manissha Shah
Qualification	:	B.Com., CA, CWA, DISA (ICA)
Current Profession	:	Counselor and Coach
Age	:	55 years
E-mail ID	:	**authormanissha@gmail.com**
City/ Country	:	**Ahmedabad, India**

Manissha Shah, academically is a Chartered Accountant as well as a Cost Accountant, with nearly 30 years of rich experience, focusing in the area of Information Systems Audit.

After many years of rich experience as a Chartered Accountant, she decided to go ahead with her burning desire and passion to create a positive change in the lives of people. She studied to be a Life Coach, a Relationship Coach, NLP Coach, Law of Attraction Coach, Master Practitioner of Graphology, Spiritual healer and many other peripheral courses. She not only has successfully transformed lives of hundreds of people in the areas of mental and emotional health and wellbeing, physical health challenges, relationship challenges, career challenges, financial challenges, but has also helped them create abundance in life.

Having very successfully, transformed cases of marital discord and those on the verge of a divorce into very beautiful marriage relationships, she decided to pen some of her thoughts, to inspire people to instill romance in their marriage.

The anthology, **"Seven LEE of Life"** is a beautifully designed collection of the Learnings, Earnings and Expectations from the lives of 108 co-authors, including me.

As human beings, we all face up and downs in life. But handling the difficult and trying situations in life is challenging, at times. A different perspective of looking at it, at times, helps ease the situation.

With the strength, power, confidence and various other values that I have learnt and earned over the years, I have made a humble effort to pen them down, with faith that they could create a positive change in someone's life.

Learning :

1. Always be in the 'GIVING' Mode, without any expectation of getting anything in return. 'Giving' could be either in monetary terms or it could be in non monetary terms (in fact, which are more valuable) – could be kindness, appreciation, gratitude, emotional support, moral support, empathy, guidance, understanding, a strong shoulder during their difficult times or any other support that could help them tide away their challenges effectively.

2. The Universe never 'gives', it always 'returns'. Whatever we get in life – good, bad or ugly, is what we have, knowingly or unknowingly given someone else in life, and the universe is returning that to us. For example: if someone has cheated you of money, you certainly have, cheated some one else either of money, trust, love or anything else, and the universe is merely returning that cheatery to you.

3. Whatever happens, happens for the best – whether we realise it soon or a few decades later. Even terrible situations can make us stronger, if we stand firm.

4. Value your relations – spend 'quality' time with your family and friends. This is something you'll treasure all your life

5. A perfectly beautiful relationship is one where two imperfect souls accept each other exactly as they are. Nobody is perfect in this world. Realise this to make each and every relationship of yours perfect.

6. People may forget what you said or did, but they will never forget the way you made them feel. Make everyone feel good.

7. Forgive others – not because it makes you feel superior, but because you value your relationships more than anything else.

Earning :

Some of the Priceless Earnings that I have earned in life, which make me feel absolutely 'wealthy' are:

1. **Beautiful Relationships:** I have been blessed with beautiful relationships be they family, friends and/or others - where Friends are Family and Family are Friends. The love, care, trust and support that I have got from them are priceless.

2. **Ability to Get up:** after every fall, more determined. Falls do not deter me from achieving my goals, infact I return stronger.

3. **Ability to Empathise:** This ability, that I have earned, has helped me get out the best in people, strengthen my bonds with them and most importantly, strengthen myself.

4. **Opportunities to be of help:** I am certainly very grateful to the Universe, for making me capable and deserving of getting umpteen opportunities to be of help and get a lovely smile on their face too.

5. **The Power to be Grateful:** Life has taught me to be grateful for anything and everything that I get in life. This power has rewarded me by helping me get out of tough situations, easily and effortlessly, most of the times.

6. **The Power to turn any Obstacle into an Opportunity:** Effect of wrong decisions during difficult times, along with the opportunity for me to be a life coach, have taught me to think effectively for a solution that every challenge always has – This is a **'Priceless Gem'** for me.

7. **Humility and Modesty:** Ups and downs in life have taught me to be more humble and modest. These values have helped wade through the storms in life, gracefully.

Expectation :

1. The power to be able to heal each and every one, whom I get connected to, whether physically or virtually, directly or indirectly, knowingly or accidentally or whichever way, and get a wonderful smile on their faces.

2. Be absolutely fit, fine and healthy, in each and every way to take up any challenge in life and fulfil it to the tee.

3. Start an NGO (Non Government Organisation) wherein marital challenges, upto divorce are either
    - Sorted out, and the couple decide to give a fresh beginning to their life OR
    - Fought out, and that too, absolutely Honestly and Diligently, with my investigating team verifying the genuiness of both the parties, fact and circumstances of the case etc. Competence of my lawyers shall be a prerequisite.

4. An opportunity to create a world, wherein everyone gives and gets lots of love and compassion, to and from everyone.

5. Opportunities to contribute as much as possible to create World Peace

6. The power to create the Power within me, to help others achieve each and every dream of theirs.

7. Leave behind a legacy of love, care, compassion and honesty.

|| ॐ ||

Mayur Ghate

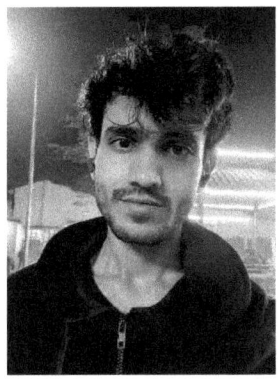

Author's Name	:	Mayur Ghate
Qualification	:	M.Sc.
Current Profession	:	Pursuing Ph.D.
Age	:	33 years
E-mail ID	:	**mayur.ghate3@gmail.com**
City/ Country	:	**Dombivli, India**

Mayur Ghate is currently pursuing his Ph.D in the field of Biotechnology at Indian Institute of Technology, Roorkee (IIT, Roorkee). He has done his Master Degrees in Biotechnology at Banaras Hindu University, Varanasi (BHU, Varanasi).

Apart from his PhD, he has enrolled in other certification courses like Neuro Linguistic Programming (NLP). Ho'Oponopono and EFT program, Handwriting analyst, Law of attraction coach.

Anthology provides a great opportunity for the persons like me who wish to write and become an author. I know and comprehend the current scenario of the society, and willing to convey my learnings and make people familiar with the truth. Through anthology, it becomes possible to reach to thousands and thousands of people and change their lives for the betterment. As this platform is the amalgamation of precious thoughts and experiences of authors, people can easily relate with their own experiences that can add value in their lives. Finally, it bestows confidence among people and motivates them to become expressive.

Learning :

1. Self-Love
2. Self-Acceptance
3. Self-worth
4. Forgiveness
5. We all are one and connected
6. We are spiritual beings
7. Listen to soul

Earning :

1. Self-acceptance
2. Health
3. Compassion for people
4. Sense of responsibility
5. Valuing the gift of life
6. Being grateful for everything
7. Releasing negative emotions everyday

Expectation :

1. Growth
2. Love and connection
3. Acceptance of balance of life
4. Contribution to the society
5. Uplifting the society
6. Enjoying and sharing all the materialistic things as human
7. Creating a bright future for my generation

|| ॐ ||

Mehul Gupta

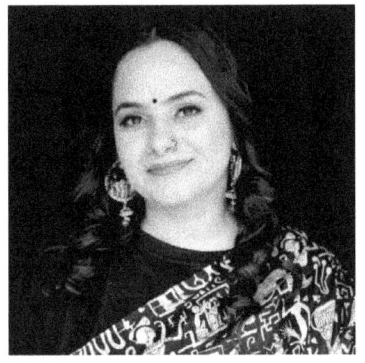

Author's Name	:	Mehul Gupta
Qualification	:	B.Com.
Current Profession	:	Smile Coach
Age	:	37 years
E-mail ID	:	**mehulgupta.8611@gmail.com**
City/ Country	:	**New Delhi, India**

Mehul Gupta is an independent woman and a dedicated smile coach, bringing joy and positivity into the lives of those she counsels. With a gentle heart and a nurturing spirit, she embodies the essence of an angel, healing people around her with compassion and kindness. Her mission is to inspire and uplift and guide others toward a happier, more fulfilled life through the power of smiles and positive energy. She believes in the transformative power of genuine connection and strives to create a ripple effect of happiness. Every smile she shares and every heart she heals is a step towards a brighter, more compassionate world. www.guptamehul.com

Mehul Gupta has the below LEEs of life :

Learning :

1. **Charge:** Be careful who you trust. Salt & Sugar look the same.
2. **Repetition:** Lessons in life will be repeated until they are learnt.
3. **Timing:** I have learned that I've a lot to learn.
4. **Be Yourself:** It sounds Simple but requires great Faith.

5. **Trust:** Our own Life has to be our message.
6. **You:** Be there for others, but never leave yourself behind
7. **At the End** of the Day, It is what it is.

Earning :

1. Your Life isn't a movie. Don't let other people write the script.
2. Choose to see the World.
3. What is your Why?
4. You will never be ready. Just start.
5. Prove them Wrong.
6. Invest in Yourself. You can afford it
7. One Day is TODAY.

Expectation :

1. Observe Accept Release Transform
2. Go the Extra mile it's never crowded.
3. Value your peace more than people's expectation.
4. Wake-up Smile and tell ypurself Today is my day.
5. There's magic on the other side of fear.
6. To go forward you have to leave something behind.
7. Certain darkness is needed to see the stars.

|| ॐ ||

Mini Baijal

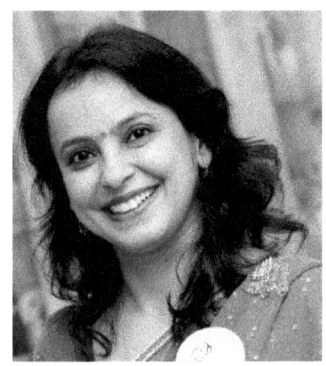

Author's Name	:	Mini Baijal
Qualification	:	B.Sc. B.Ed with PG Diploma in Management
Current Profession	:	Headmistress in a Private School
Age	:	52 Years
E-mail ID	:	**minikbaijal@gmail.com**
City/ Country	:	**Gurgaon, India**

Mini Baijal is the Headmistress of a renowned private school in Gurgaon. She is in the field of education for more than 22 years. She is a passionate educator who bagged **'School Spirit Award'** in 2018 and **'Best Teacher Award'** twice in 2019 and 2020. She was honored with **'District Performance Excellence Award'** 2019-20 by Science Olympiad Foundation. She was also conferred with **'Rotary District 3011 Excellence Award'** and a certificate of achievement for significant contribution at Sakshar. Her effort of imparting knowledge to the 21st Century Learners was appreciated and was felicitated at the Rotary Annual Award ceremony on 5 September 2023.

I believe that whatever happens, it happens for good. Life is not smooth for everyone. It is always good to accept whatever comes in our life then there will be less of suffering. Every incident gives us happiness or learning. Our good deeds will give happiness to us too. Our spiritual earnings will improve the quality of our life. Some people consider excess of materialistic things as their wealth but the true wealth is actually the peace of mind. Expectations are the beliefs that something will happen. Like others, I do have some expectations from my life. I understand that our expectations give happiness if fulfilled but we get learning if they are not fulfilled. They push us towards our goal and direct our behaviour. My understanding about **LEEs** of Life –

Learning :

1. **Joyfulness** - Life is very short. Don't complain for what you don't have but enjoy what you have.

2. **Spiritual Wellbeing** - I am responsible for my happiness. No one can disturb my mental peace unless I allow them to do so.

3. **Grace and Gratitude** - I have received what I have given. If I will spread happiness I will receive happiness, if I will give hatred how I can expect love.

4. **Temperance** - People around me are not my puppets. They do have their choices and opinions.

5. **Being Positive** - One should stay positive all the time. It attracts positivity. If we keep complaining or use bad words we will attract negativity.

6. **Faith** - Whatever belongs to me will come to me sooner or later. If something does not belong to me, it will never be mine or stay with me.

7. **Self-Love** - The good work done is always appreciated and recognised by everyone. Keep doing good, you need not justify yourself.

Earning :

1. **Gratitude** - My gratitude to almighty for blessing me with a respectable and healthy life.

2. **Patience** - I am fortunate to have the blessings of my parents who have taught me patience and perseverance.

3. **Virtuous** - I have got a very loving and caring family which means that I must have done something good in my life.

4. **Thankfulness** - I am blessed to have a home, family and a good job.

5. **Humility** - I am an educationist and I have received so much love and affection from my students.

6. **Fortitude** – I can deal with difficult and painful situations while keeping my calm and composure.

7. **Resilience** - Being able to evolve as a better version of myself is my spiritual earning.

Expectation :

1. **Dedication** - I should be able to justify my being and my role on this mother earth.

2. **Socially responsible** - I should be able to give back to the society.

3. **Dutiful** - I should be able to make my parents proud of me.

4. **Commitment** - I am a mother, a teacher and a mentor. I need to justify all these roles too.

5. **My Country My Pride** - I want to visit all parts of my country India.

6. **To be Philanthropist** - Life should give me an opportunity to open a school for underprivileged children.

7. **Self-Discipline** - I want to be a learner throughout my life. I pray to almighty to allow me to learn and try new thing during this journey of my life.

॥ ॐ ॥

Neelam Khemani

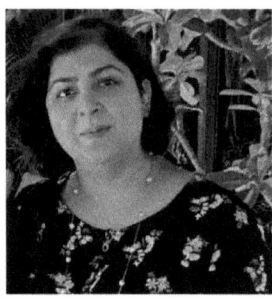

Author's Name	:	Neelam Khemani
Qualification	:	M.B.A
Current Profession	:	Consultant
Age	:	46 Years
E-mail ID	:	...
City/ Country	:	**Hyderabad, India**

Neelam Khemani has done her MBA in Finance. She has 18+ years' experience of Product Management and Operations in the areas of Business Research & Analysis in India and U.S. as well. She is a mother of a beautiful girl and a nurturer. She loves movies and music on long drive!

I am sharing few things that life has taught over the years of ups and downs, and more so the lowest times of my life where I went numb / dead. I realize now that things could have been dealt differently and better. This revelation and growth, of course came from a lot of support from family and friends and various other people who touched my life.

Learning :

1. **Acceptance**: we need to allow people be who they are and accept them while drawing your boundaries, else be prepared for things to fall apart.

2. **Ease**: We need to be adaptable to the changes life and people bring with them and ensure there is an ease with which life can flow without clenching on to thoughts/ beliefs.

3. **Feel your feelings**: We are all allowed to feel sad / angry / bad / mourn / be happy / excited…but ensure you regulate and centre yourself without becoming a negative and a complaining person.

4. **Birds eye view**: Life / people / situations need to be looked at from a neutral perspective to be able to not get emotionally entangled and lose our rational to face / resolve it.
5. **Constant evolution**: it is key to continually evolve intellectually, emotionally and spiritually or ready to drown in stagnancy. Trauma is no excuse to play dead.
6. **Gratitude**: Always have gratitude for what is going alright in your life…. else even that might just go away like everything else!
7. **Never Compare:** If you are made to stand in a circle and exchange your life happiness or issues with anyone? Would you? Most say No and hence never compare.

Earning:

1. **Empath:** Being a hardcore empath has helped me understand and help so many people. Will always be grateful to life for giving me this quality.
2. **Pay it forward:** my biggest learning and earning in this lifetime is to be able to pay it forward in whichever way I can.
3. **My friendships:** unconditional love and acceptance that I able to give to friends around me and their love in return
4. **Non-judgemental:** I let anyone be without judging them or categorizing/labelling them. Allows me to sleep in peace without negativity.
5. **Thrive on self-improvement:** Be it intellectual, emotional maturity and spiritually - this is my legacy that I know I will leave behind with pride
6. **My graceful ability** to handle the adversities of life and continual learnings from it and evolving from it.
7. **What you see/ hear is what you get.** I live life without playing games or lying to myself/ others /Universe. Else, we are all going to get entangled in it.

Expectation:

1. **Unconditional love** and acceptance is something I hope this lifetime will help me with
2. **Financial growth** and independence is what I am requesting the Universe
3. **Every cell in harmony** – whether or not I get what I want – is the end goal / expectation from myself
4. **Faith** – Unwavering faith is something I want to work on
5. **Ability to assimilate** as much knowledge / wisdom in this lifetime
6. **Ease in the flow of life** - of friendships, progress, finances, wisdom, composure, etc
7. I need to help and touch as many lives as I can before I leave this planet

|| ॐ ||

Neena Puri Nagpal

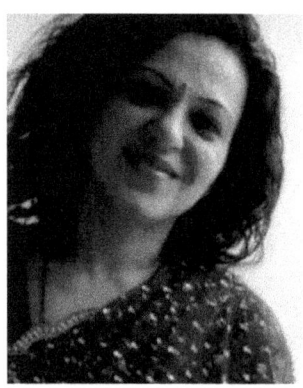

Author's Name	:	Neena Puri Nagpal
Qualification	:	MBA (Finance)
Current Profession	:	Director, Private Banking
Age	:	46 years
E-mail ID	:	**neenapuri@yahoo.com**
City/ Country	:	**Gurugram, India**

Neena Puri Nagpal is a BFSI professional with 17 years of Indian and Offshore market experience. Presently working as Director with India's leading bank. She is learner for life, always seeking new experiences and always embracing new opportunities. She is an incredible multi – tasker, someone who always strives for excellence in all domains, be it professional or personal. Most of all, she firmly believes in hard work – and that there's nothing in the world that cannot be achieved with hard work and patience. She is doting mother of two adorable kids, who loves a simple and wholesome living – a living that prioritizes self-care and mental health while balancing all other aspects of life

The topic essentially wants us to pause and reflect on whatever life experiences have taught us so far. The key episodes of life and what we make of those determine the course of our lives, our relationships, our emotional and happiness quotient. Likewise, our life journey too forms expectations that we have from ourselves and from others, from our inner circle and other layers. While it is commonly believed that expectation is the sure door for disappointments. But what is life without expectations. I'd rather work on being stoic towards outcomes of those expectations, but keep myself real by having expectations, for life certainly is give and take. Lastly, with so much effort that we put in, there certainly are earnings - tangibles as well as intangibles. Money is indispensable; things money can't buy remain core to our being.

This is a classic traditional approach to me leading my life and absorbing modern and evolving concepts that are in synchronization to my fabric are my LEE.

Learning :

1. **Balance** - The path that leads to all destinations is the middle path.
2. **Self-Love** - Priorities yourself and practice physical, mental, emotional, spiritual self-care. It's not being selfish.
3. **Inside Out** - You can give others what you have. If you have happiness inside you, only then, you shall be able to spread happiness.
4. **Personal Growth** - The capacity to learn is a gift, the ability to learn is a skill and the willingness to learn is a choice. Exercise that choice.
5. **Change** - Accepting change allows for adaptation, resilience and opportunity for transformative experiences.
6. **Lock the bulls by its horns** - Whether internal crisis or external, whether internal dilemma or external, confront. Denial will not lead to solution, will only prolong misery and unhappiness.
7. **Nucleus of love** - For small creatures such as us, the vastness is bearable only through love.

Earning :

1. **Wholesome life** - Family, friends, career, self-awareness-important ingredients for a wholesome life.
2. **Thick skinned** - honed an ability to cut through noise to pursue what matters most to me.
3. **Simplicity** - Open, direct, soulful communication avoiding mind games.
4. **Choose being wise over street smart** - If long term relationships matter, becoming wise is a great choice.
5. **Maturity** - Ability to handle uncertainty
6. **Respond, don't react** - don't take actions of other people Striving to keep bridges firm, never burn them.
7. **Building bridges** -Old connections are as important as new ones. Build bridges, never burn them.

Expectation :

1. **Best things in life are free** - Figuring out my mojo is constant work in progress.
2. **Money is still important** - Expect myself to be able to fulfill needs and wants of my near and dear ones, and of my own.
3. **Bloodline** - Family is not always blood. Look out for meaningful connections outside of family and cultivate them equally passionately.

4. **Time** - Time heals. Give time the time to heal.

5. **Battlefront** - Choose your battles wisely.

6. **Meaning** - Go after what it is that creates meaning in your life and then trust yourself to handle the stress that follows.

7. **Love** - Love is our true destiny. We don't find the meaning of our life by ourselves alone; we find it with another.

|| ॐ ||

Neetu A Beel

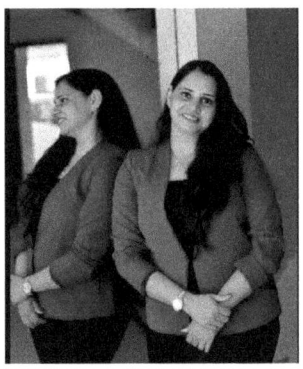

Author's Name	:	Neetu A Beel
Qualification	:	B.Com.
Current Profession	:	Numerologist, Graphologist
Age	:	42 Years
E-mail ID	:	accessvibrations@gmail.com
City/ Country	:	**Kolkata, India**

Neetu A Beel is a distinguished Numerologist and Graphologist with over 12 years of experience, dedicated to helping individuals transform their lives. As a certified Bach Flower therapist, she specializes in healing emotional wounds that often manifest as physical ailments.

Neetu's expertise extends to Past Life Regression therapy, guiding people to uncover the hidden roots of their present challenges. Her mission is to empower others with knowledge of the unseen forces that shape their lives, offering profound insights into the invisible but powerful energies that influence our existence. Neetu is passionate about educating and uplifting people, helping them unlock their full potential and lead a more balanced, harmonious life.

While writing about the **'Seven LEE of Life'**, I found myself deeply connected with my inner self, reflecting on the profound gratitude I feel. We are here on Earth not just to live but to experience, evolve and grow. Human evolution is not merely physical; it encompasses the soul's journey and the lessons we are destined to learn. The true essence of life is the wisdom we acquire, the knowledge we earn, and the growth we achieve—all of which we carry with us into the next lifetime. The learning and spiritual wealth that truly define our journey, guiding us toward our higher purpose, I am deeply thankful for every lesson life has learnt, each one shaping my path in unique and beautiful ways. These experiences have molded me, contributing to the continuous evolution of my soul.

Learning :

1. **Happiness:** happiness is always a choice
2. **Help everyone:** it will come back to you
3. **Karma:** what goes around, comes around
4. **Everything is interconnected:** our past present and future
5. **Live life:** The moments you love, laugh and learn, are the moment you live life
6. **There is no coincidence:** everything happens for a reason
7. **Trust:** if god is breaking you, he is making you

Earning :

1. My children, my biggest wealth
2. My husband, my life partner is my guide for life
3. My knowledge, it changed me completely
4. My circle, people around me, my family my friends are very important for me
5. My personality, my courage and my confident
6. My understanding and helping nature
7. My intuition, always helped me

Expectation :

1. Want to travel around the world
2. My children will become a good human being
3. Want to start NGO for orphan kids and old people
4. Want to remove all the garbage from the mother earth
5. Want to plant more trees and clean the lakes and rivers
6. Want to be fit and healthy both mentally and physically
7. Want to create multiple source of income and help other people to earn

|| ॐ ||

Neha Piyush Nashine

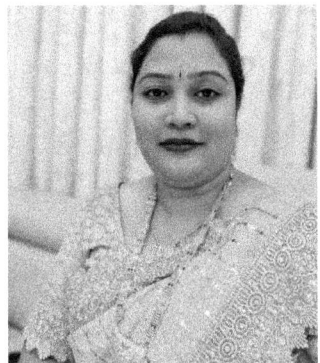

Author's Name	:	Neha Piyush Nashine
Qualification	:	Bachelor in Arts
Current Profession	:	Vastu Consultant, Numerologist, Tarot Card Reader, Author and Electrical Contractor
		▪ Proprietor - Shivansh Electrical and Infra Works
		▪ Director - Kulamama Resorts Pvt. Ltd.
Age	:	35 Years
E-mail ID	:	**npnashine@gmail.com**
City/ Country	:	**Nagpur, India**

Mrs. Neha Piyush Nashine is an Entrepreneur, Vastu Expert, Numerologist and Tarot Card Reader. She is also in Hospitality Business Director at Kulamama Resorts Pvt. Ltd. and A Proprietor at Shivansh Electrical & Infra Works makes her an independent woman. She strongly believes in hard work and is an optimistic person always ready to learn with a positive attitude spirituality is her strength.

Neha has the below LEEs of life :

L for Learning is a comprehensive life-long important process, learning is the innate nature of human being. Every day every person keeps collecting new experiences in his life, These new experiences increase and modify a person's behavior, that is why these experiences and their use are called learning. Learning new understanding, knowledge, behavior, skills, values, attitudes and primary level receiving process. This Process of Larning abilities are in Humans and animals.

E for Earning, Income is the amount of money you earn from doing some Work.

However, money received from investment can also be called income. A company's earnings, in simple words, are its profits. The money received by selling Product or service is called earning. Subtract all the costs of producing the product or service and that's your income. Of course, the details of accounting become much more complex. But earnings always show how much money a company or individual makes after deducting its costs.

E for Expectation, Hope Expectation is a strong belief something will happen or it will happen like this, Our expectations more than anything else determine our reality And our expectations also affect the people around us. In a self-prophecy people can flood or fall depending on our expectation and belief on.

Learning :

1. Vastu Shastra
2. Numerology
3. Tarot Card Reading
4. Resort Business
5. Housewife
6. Relegious
7. Palmistry

Earning :

1. Money, Name and Fame
2. Confidence
3. Earn Respect and Fame
4. Name, Fame & Money
5. Knowledge of Sanatan Dharm
6. Respect
7. Finding Solution for Peoples Problem.

Expectation :

1. To grow more to help people
2. To gain more knowledge and become a famous numerologist
3. Finding the solution of human problem
4. Get closer to God
5. Need respect from family members

6. To be the best in my profession
7. To do good something for Nation

॥ ॐ ॥

Nidhi Chugh

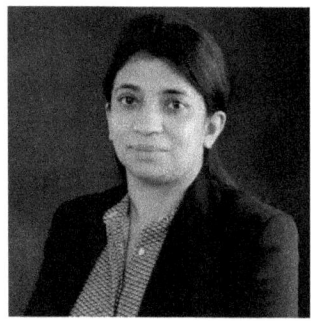

Author's Name	:	Nidhi Chugh
Qualification	:	B.A. English (Hons), Certified Graphologist
Current Profession	:	Consultant, Numerologist, Astro-Vastu Expert and Logo Designer
Age	:	49 years
E-mail ID	:	**numerologistnidhichugh@gmail.com**
City/ Country	:	**Gurgaon, India**

Nidhi Chugh is a self-motivated and hard-working individual who has made a significant mark in the fields of graphology, numerology and Vaastu. She is a Certified Graphologist specializing in handwriting and signature analysis. In 2011, she completed her advanced course in graphology from the International School of Handwriting Analysis (ISHA USA, California). Additionally, she undertook an advanced course from Power of Handwriting in India and currently serves as the Delhi NCR head of the organization.

Nidhi's extensive experience includes conducting workshops on personality development through handwriting in schools and corporate offices. She has also worked in the HR departments of several offices abroad, focusing on recruitment processes. Her knowledge in Vaastu, combined with her skills in numerology and graphology, allows her to assist individuals in overcoming a range of challenges, including delays in marriage, relationship issues, court cases, and financial difficulties.

For corporate clients, Nidhi acts as a solution provider, helping organizations recruit the right personnel through her expertise in numerology and graphology. She also works to balance the energies within corporate premises, contributing to a harmonious work environment. Nidhi offers consultations both online and offline, having successfully completed over 5,000 cases that include homes, factories and commercial establishments.

Nidhi Chugh has the below LEEs of life :

Learning :

1. **Curiosity:** The desire to learn new things about one's environment and ask many questions. Exploring and wondering are what characterise a curious individual.

2. **Discovery:** The stage that involves the development of earlier-held ideas based on the simulation to find new things and ask questions. It's also the stage when one investigates sites, pieces of information, or geometric forms.

3. **Understanding:** Higher levels of knowledge are provided by grasping the meaning of concepts and ideas proficiently enough to relate and comprehend their relationships.

4. **Retention:** This, in most cases, refers to the ability to store knowledge and retrieve it when needed in the future.

5. **Reflection:** Reviewing previously passed learning events to learn something from them. It also brings out the aspect of maturity.

6. **Application:** This can refer to utilising previously learned knowledge in practical situations to address problems or add value.

7. **Adaptability:** Knowing one's ability and adjusting one's expectations and learning styles when presented with new ideas.

Earning :

1. **Value:** The definition of value regards worth, which, in this case, connects more to how one's work is delivered than to how much one can earn.

2. **Service:** Enriching communities through helping others creates bonds and brings people together.

3. **Integrity:** Being guided by moral principles in carrying out one's work to inspire trust and respect in a person or to relationships of trust to vision.

4. **Contribution:** The idea of taking action and doing something that adds value to the society or a community and better the society or the community as a whole.

5. **Gratitude:** is the virtue that comes from recognising and appreciating what one has at hand or what can be accessed externally, making it easy and obligated to work to earn.

6. **Empowerment:** Helping other people control their own lives and make choices and decisions that are helpful for them in many aspects, such as education or business.

7. **Sustainability:** Earning through the available opportunities while involving respect for the resources and doing so for the sake of the coming generations and the future.

Expectation :

1. **Anticipation:** This is the excitement and eagerness experienced when someone feels that a certain time or event will come.

2. **Standards** refer to the set of criteria, specifications, rules, or principles that are used as the basis for performance or evaluation.

3. **Perception:** The act of seeing, hearing, and understanding, which, in turn, helps in the formulation of expectations that a person possesses upon others or different outcomes.

4. **Disappointment:** I think it refers to the sense of grief and annoyance experienced when a person is unable to achieve what they hoped for.

5. **Assumption:** This is often the case when a person has some expectation in relation to the other party's action but does not check or validate whether their action was indeed the case.

6. **Reality:** In short it is what exists or the state of things as they actually are contrary to what a person may expect.

7. **Flexibility** refers to the readiness, willingness or ability to shift goals in relation to the existing conditions or new information to aid in one's progress.

|| ॐ ||

Nimishaa Mathur

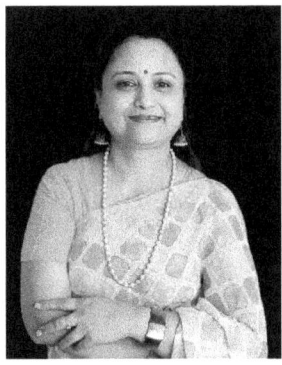

Author's Name	:	Nimishaa Mathur
Qualification	:	M.Sc. (Chemistry), B.Ed.
Current Profession	:	CXO @ Home
Age	:	42 years
E-mail ID	:	…
City/ Country	:	**New Delhi, India**

Mrs Nimishaa Mathur is working as a full-time **Home Manager**. She is passionate for wandering, cooking, gardening and rhythmically tapping the floor. She is enthusiastic about social service and counselling. She is an empathetic listener and vocal on social issues. She is qualified as a Trained Teacher (B.Ed.) and M.Sc. in Chemistry with a long teaching experience.

Nimishaa has the below LEEs of life :

Learning :

1. **Never Over Commit:** Over commitment leads to unhealthy and weak relations. Promise only which you can deliver

2. **Learn to Say No:** It is perfectly fine to say No if you are not comfortable or disagree. One thing to remember while saying No is it should not be blunt or rude

3. **Be Assertive:** Stand for your rights. No one else is going to do this for you.

4. **Know your Worth:** Accept yourself, love yourself and be grounded as a person who you are.

5. **Acceptance:** Acceptance to people, situation and circumstances gives you the courage to fight back and overcome the situation.

6. **Gratitude:** Being grateful connects you to the energy that brings you more of what you have.

7. **Be Compassionate:** We as souls are travellers in this world and we do not know what pain the other soul might have faced through these journeys so be kind and treat people generously.

Earning :

1. **Happily Married:** Had a tough walk through but my positive efforts made me a happily married woman.

2. **Social Circle:** I have a good friend circle with positive mindset and helping attitude.

3. **Intellect:** Being vocal and participative on social issues i became eloquent and visionary.

4. **Empathic listener:** My friends call me an empathic listener as I can hear them for hours. They share their pain, sorrow as I understand the depth of their words.

5. **Motivator and Counsellor:** I keep motivating my friends and family to achieve their goals of life and if stuck somewhere they love to get counselling from me.

6. **Passionate Cook:** Proud journey of not even know to make tea to a home Chef running a YouTube channel and participant of a National cooking competition.

7. **Travel Takeaways:** Travelled to various exotic as well as offbeat places and witnessed different cultures.

Expectation :

1. **Food Joint:** I want to own a famous food joint.

2. **Travel:** I want to travel and explore the beauty of this world. I want to be in the lap of nature.

3. **Big happy family:** I want to have a big family with everyone sharing love and feelings with each other and living peacefully and United.

4. **Second Inning:** I want to live my second inning of life where everyone around me feels happy and proud to be associated with me.

5. **Author:** I want to become a renowned author. I want to jot down my ideas on counselling and peaceful life path where we respect each other's feelings.

6. **Best Mother in Law:** I want to turn out to be best mom in law where I will always support, understand, love and care my daughter in laws.

7. **Old Age Home:** I want to run a old age home where people who are being disowned by their family are being taken care off.

|| ॐ ||

Nitender Mann

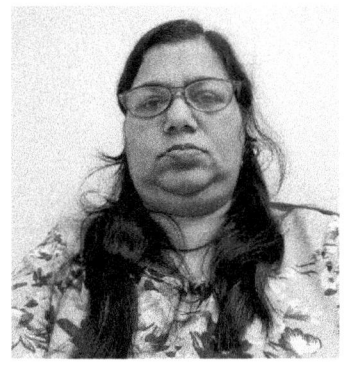

Author's Name	:	Nitender Mann
Qualification	:	B. Ed,, M.A.
Current Profession	:	Consultant and Counselor
Age	:	46 years
E-mail ID	:	**nitendermann@gmail.com**
City/ Country	:	**Toronto, Canada**

Nitender Mann is a budding Author and Certified Astro-Numerologist and Tarot Card Reader. She has done his Bachelor of Education in English and Economics. She has also done her Master Degree in Economics. She had worked more than 15 years as a teacher in reputed school in Punjab, India as well as in Canada. Now she is working in an accounting and insurance office as well as practicing in Occult Sciences.

Life is a complex and dynamic journey in which we keep on learning since our birth. While learning we keep on growing and doing self improvement. While learning new things in life, we also keep on earning not only financially but in all aspects of life and with these learning and earning from life we have expectations like what other things we have to do in our life. Expectation from our life can sometimes help in achieving goals but other times it also gives you disappointment and frustration. I have also learned ,earned many things from life and also have expectations from life,

Learning :

1. **Accept the change -** I learned that life is unpredictable and uncertain.So we should always adapt to learn the changes that life gives you.

2. **Forgive and let it Go** - We should also learn to forgive others for the mistakes they have made even if they have hurt you a lot.
3. **Keep on trying** - We should also keep on trying in spite of failures.Even you fail in certain areas of life we should never give up .Remember to keep on trying until you achieve success.
4. **Learn to give Gratitude and Appreciation** - We should always give gratitude to the persons in your life who have given you support in times of need,never forget those people in life,And also give appreciation to those who are working hard to make your life beautiful.
5. **Always be Curious** - You should always be in a mode of learning, We should always keep on learning.Continuous learning in life helps us to grow more for the whole life.
6. **Learn to take responsibility** - Always take the responsibilities of your own actions and decisions.Taking responsibilities leads to growth and self-awareness.
7. **Listen to your heart** - Always listen to your heart means do not ignore your interest and passion .By listening to your heart it will give us a lot of joy and fulfillment from inner self.

Earning :

1. **Connections** - I learned to make a lot of connections means a lot of relationships with families ,friends and community ties .
2. **Knowledge** - Through continuous learning, I have had the opportunity to gain a lot of knowledge which has been quite instrumental in my personal and professional growth.
3. **Experience** - I have gathered valuable life experiences that have shaped my view and wisdom.I learned lot of modalities in the field of occult science,
4. **Self-Confidence** - I have learned to overcome challenges that come my way and thus be confident and believe in my abilities.
5. **Respect** - I have earned a lot of respect from others by the fact that I always give respect to others so that in return I also get the respect.I always gives others good advice.
6. **Gratitude** - I've developed a deep sense of appreciation for the kinds of people and opportunities that have made my life richer.
7. **Financial Stability** - I must admit that, through hard work and perseverance, I have obtained financial stability to follow my passions.

Expectation :

1. **Growth:** I am supposed to keep on growing and changing all through my life in personal ,spiritual and professional aspects.
2. **Fulfillment:** I expect to be able to find fulfillment in that which I am doing since I follow my passion.
3. **Balance:** I will ensure that I achieve a healthy work-life balance whereby I have time for personal and professional life.

4. **Happiness:** It's supposed to bring happiness if I can actually do what I am passionate about and be true to myself.

5. **Contribution:** I look forward to being able to contribute more meaningfully to society with my skills and knowledge in the field of occult by helping other people.

6. **Resilience:** Yes, I do expect to build my resilience by standing up before challenging situations and persevering.

7. **Legacy:** It is my expectation to be able to leave behind along last impact that will continue affecting others even when I am gone.

|| ॐ ||

Om Prakash Priyadarshi

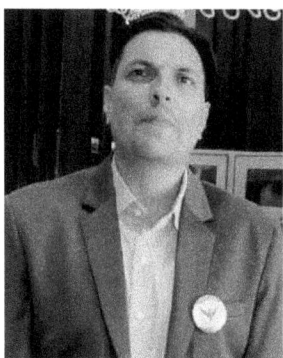

Author's Name	:	Om Prakash Priyadarshi
Qualification	:	M.A, LLB, PGDBM, PGDLL
Current Profession	:	Realtor, Film maker, Human Behavior Expert, Inner Health Physician in handwriting, Professional Grapho Therapist Analyst & Coach
Age	:	38 years
E-mail ID	:	Omprakashpriyadarshi612@gmail.com
City/ Country	:	Noida, India

Om Prakash Priyadarshi is Real Estate Business Owner and also associated with an internationally renowned real estate company Exp Realty. He is Certified Professional Handwriting Analyst, Inner Physician health in Handwriting & Professional Grapho-therapist Analyst from international council of Graphologist. He is also Certified in Occult Mastery program. He has done LLB, Master Degrees in politics, Post graduate diploma in business management in Human resources management and post graduate diploma in Labor Laws. He had worked more than 15 years in Central government in different locations of India.

He is also aspiring Film maker, Actor and Director working on different Assignments. As realtor and digital expert helping Businesses in team building and digital automation.

Om Prakash Priyadarshi is also Human behavior expert. He strongly believes that the parents and the teachers can become "Changemaker" of our current education system to make India proud to become land of education, along with he helps students of age group 11 years and above to solving their academic issues, emotional issues, financial challenges & different other challenges of study.

The **'Seven LEE of Life'** anthology brings together three key areas—Learning, Earning and Expectation—to guide us toward a fulfilling life. In *Learning*, we explore the power of believing in ourselves, sharing our unique stories, practicing self-care, and finding our voice. It's about growing from within. *Earning* looks at how we gain recognition, build wealth, and contribute to society, while also mentoring others and helping in times of need. It's not just about money—it's about making a positive impact. Finally, *Expectation* focuses on our bigger dreams: creating peace, protecting the planet, caring for the elderly and orphans, and ensuring happiness and financial security for future generations. Together, these seven aspects show how we can live a balanced, meaningful life, full of purpose and kindness.

Learning :

1. Believe in yourself, anything is possible.
2. Every human story is unique so we should tell it with pride.
3. Self-care is not selfish, it's essential.
4. Our Voice matters.
5. Forgiveness is true kindness and gratitude to that person.
6. We should have passion-driven life.
7. Time will automatically manage if we manage our habits.

Earning :

1. Public recognition
2. My book and author journey
3. Contribution to my physical and wealth part of my life.
4. Trust
5. Help in disaster relief
6. Mentorship to others
7. Plantation

Expectation :

1. Peace for humanity
2. Save this earth to environment pollution
3. At least one old age home.
4. At least one orphanage.
5. At least one animal and bird habitat center

6. Financial freedom to my next generation
7. Happiness for every creature on the earth.

॥ ॐ ॥

Pooja Gulati

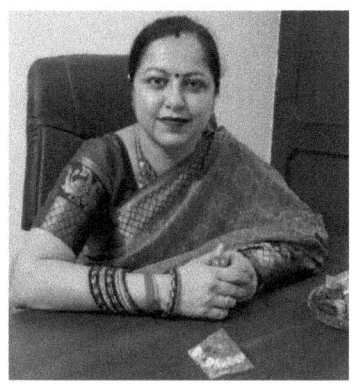

Author's Name	:	Pooja Gulati
Qualification	:	M.A., B.Ed.
Current Profession	:	Consultant, Numerologist, Vastu Expert, Crystal Healer, Switch Word Expert, Pendulum Dowser
Age	:	44 years
E-mail ID	:	**27poojagulati27@gmail.com**
City/ Country	:	**Meerut, India**

Pooja Gulati is a renowned and Certified Numerologist. She has done her B.Ed. and Master Degree in Arts and completed all her education from Pune University. She has worked as a teacher in a renowned school in Meerut for 10 years and is now working for the upliftment of people and helping them release their problems through numerology and other sciences of occult. She uses different techniques and remedies through switch words, crystals, healing numbers, pendulum dowsing, aromatherapy, color therapy, bachflowers to heal people.

Life is not only a bed of roses, it also has thorns in it. Both teach us something. We get new experiences, meet new people every moment and through our own experiences we learn ,expect and also earn from life. In this anthology we are talking about Seven LEE of Life. What we Learn, Earn and Expect from life. It is a journey of discovery, connection and evolution.

Learning :

1. Learn to say NO
2. Money is very important

3. We can't please everyone
4. Health is a valuable treasure
5. Focus on working smarter than harder
6. You are stronger than you think
7. All problems have solutions

Earning :
1. Respect
2. Happiness
3. Love
4. Good Friends
5. Good Family
6. Reputation
7. Never give up attitude

Expectations :
1. Luxuries
2. To be best in my field
3. Success
4. Healthy Body
5. Healthy Mind
6. Travel around the world
7. Children should be successful

|| ॐ ||

Pooja Saxena

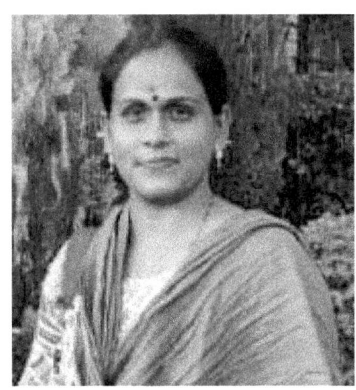

Author's Name	:	Pooja Saxena
Qualification	:	M.A.
Current Profession	:	Home Maker
Age	:	34 years
E-mail ID	:	…
City/ Country	:	**Bareilly (U.P), India**

Pooja Saxena is a dedicated individual lady, who has spent her total 10+ years of working along with shaping young minds as a teacher. After a successful career in education, she married into a joint family and she embraced the role of a homemaker, where her creativity and passion continue to thrive.

As a loving mother to a little angel, Pooja finds joy in nurturing her family, while exploring her talents in the kitchen as a passionate cook. In addition to her culinary skills, she has mastered the art of weaving and stitching, crafting various types of clothes with precision and care.

Pooja's journey reflects her commitment to both i.e. family and personal growth, blending her diverse skills with love, care and creativity.

In my understanding, the **'Seven LEE of Life'** represents a meaningful framework for navigating different stages of life. The first alphabet "L" stands for **Learning**—a lifelong process that shapes our growth and understanding. Whether through formal education or life experiences, learning is the foundation. The second alphabet "E" is for **Earning**, which comes from our efforts and hard work. It is not just about money but also about earning respect, love, and fulfillment. The third alphabet "E"

stands for **Expectation**—a double-edged sword. Managing expectations, whether from ourselves or others, is crucial to finding balance and contentment in life.

Learning :

1. **Curiosity :** Learning begins with a natural desire to explore and understand the world around us.
2. **Experience :** Life's lessons often come from real-life situations that shape our perspectives and skills.
3. **Adaptability :** Embracing change and being open to new ideas enhances our ability to learn and grow.
4. **Reflection :** Taking time to reflect on experiences helps us internalize lessons and make better decisions in the future.
5. **Mentorship :** Learning from others through mentorship can provide valuable insights and guidance on our journey.
6. **Persistence :** Overcoming challenges and staying committed to learning is key to achieving personal and professional growth.
7. **Lifelong Journey :** Learning is a continuous process that enriches our lives and prepares us for new opportunities and experiences.

Earning :

1. **Value Creation :** Earning involves creating value for others, whether through products, services, or ideas.
2. **Skill Development :** Investing in personal skills and knowledge enhances our ability to earn and succeed.
3. **Work-Life Balance :** Achieving a balance between professional and personal life is essential for sustainable earning.
4. **Networking :** Building relationships and connections can open doors to new opportunities and collaborations.
5. **Financial Literacy :** Understanding finances, investments, and savings is crucial for effective earning and wealth management.
6. **Purposeful Work :** Engaging in work that aligns with personal values brings fulfillment and deeper satisfaction in earning.
7. **Giving Back :** Earning is not just about financial gain; contributing to the community enriches both our lives and those of others.

Expectation :

1. **Love :** Earning through love involves nurturing relationships that bring joy and support to our lives.

2. **Trust :** Building trust with others creates a foundation for meaningful connections and collaborative success.

3. **Respect :** Earning respect through integrity and kindness enhances our reputation and fosters positive interactions.

4. **Gratitude :** Expressing gratitude for what we receive encourages a cycle of abundance and generosity.

5. **Empathy :** Understanding others' perspectives allows us to earn their trust and loyalty, enriching our relationships.

6. **Support :** Offering support to others creates a community where everyone can thrive and succeed together.

7. **Blessings :** Recognizing and appreciating the blessings in our lives deepens our sense of fulfillment and purpose in earning.

|| ॐ ||

Pragya Sharma

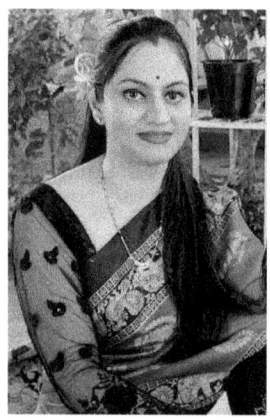

Author's Name	:	Pragya Sharma
Qualification	:	BJMC, MJMC, B.Ed., Certified Jolly Phonics Teacher
Current Profession	:	Homemaker
Age	:	32
Email id	:	sharma.pragya02@gmail.com
City/Country	:	Noida, India

Pragya Sharma has done her Master Degree in Mass Communication, Bachelor's Degree in Education and she is also a certified Jolly Phonics Teacher. She had worked with the entertainment section of one of the most renowned newspapers in India. She has also worked for more than 2 years as content writer for the magazine wherein she used to interview African Diplomats. Pragya had also worked as a primary teacher in the school.

Life has so much to offer you only if you are ready to grab it

Life is just a roller coaster of everyday adventures

They say when life gives you lemon make a lemonade out of it which is a perfect way of deceiving problems. Life is never easy for anyone; it depends on our strength to endure the difficult time. It is the greatest teacher and teaches you to be the strongest and thrive in this ever-growing world.

Here are my 'Seven LEE of Life', which I have learnt till now.

Learning :

1. **Be Calm** in every situation no matter what come may as you cannot let your anger decide what you do or what you don't.
2. Always carry a **positive mindset**.
3. **Self-love and kind**ness are very important for growth.
4. **Say no** to things which you don't like as it is your life and only you have the right to make decisions.
5. **Accept your mistakes** and learn from them.
6. **Be patient**, never give up hope and keep on trying even if you fail.
7. **Believe in yourself** as you are the hero of your own life.

These learnings have made me gain/ real earnings as well which are as follows:

Earning :

1. I feel more **happier and healthier**.
2. I am **more grateful** for the things I have rather than cribbing about what I don't have.
3. I feel more **positivity** around me.
4. I am able to take good care of my family.
5. I feel **motivated** to achieve higher success be it professionally or personally.
6. I have started enjoying significant people and achievements in my life.
7. Last but not the least I am working to be **more confident**.

Expectation :

As far as the expectations are concerned precisely I have none because the expectation is the root of all distress. We humans can only work on ourselves to make our lives a balanced one.

|| ॐ ||

Priyaa Chauhan

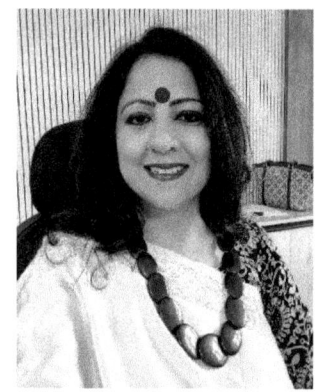

Author's Name	:	Priyaa Chauhan
Qualification	:	M.A. B.Ed.
Current Profession	:	Principal
Age	:	46 years
E-mail ID	:	...
City/ Country	:	**Gurgaon, India**

Mrs. Priyaa Chauhan, who is the Principal of G.D.Goenka Public School, is a distinguished figure in the field of education, boasting over two decades of experience. Her expertise stems from a robust academic background, holding postgraduate degrees in English & History, alongside a professional qualification in Education. Her illustrious career began at Amity International School, where she excelled as a teacher before ascending to various leadership positions in esteemed institutions across Gurgaon, including K.R.Mangalam, Lotus Valley, Shalom Hills, Laburnum School, The Pine Crest School and Mount Olympus School. Her dedication and talent have been evident throughout her journey, as she continuously strives to enhance the educational experience and nurture the minds of her students.

She has brought laurels to the schools she lead leading by winning various awards in the field of education, for an instance Award for best innovative school, Best Pre-school Award, Best school with happiness quotient and many more. Mrs Chauhan is leading the school with her vision, dedication, and passion for education. Her reputation for fostering a positive learning environment and commitment to academic excellence is truly inspiring.

In my journey of personal growth and fulfilment, I strive to embody several key principles. Gratitude guides me, reminding me that by giving generously, I often receive abundantly in return. Continuous self-improvement is a cornerstone of my life, as I believe that personal development is an ongoing process.

In terms of what I earn, my family stands as my greatest treasure, and I am profoundly grateful for the blessings I receive from those around me. My friends, though few, are precious and irreplaceable.

The positive impact I make on my students and colleagues is a source of deep satisfaction, as is the spiritual alignment that keeps me grounded and motivated. Life's varied experiences and the confidence I have in myself further enrich my journey.

Learning :

1. **Gratitude:** By giving more, you often receive more in return.
2. **Continuous Improvement:** Self-improvement is a lifelong journey with no end.
3. **Self-Assessment:** Those who cannot evaluate their own strengths and weaknesses are likely to lag behind.
4. **Health:** Prioritize health as the most crucial aspect of life.
5. **Patience:** Cultivating patience can lead to great opportunities and growth.
6. **Disposable Nature:** Recognize that you may be perceived as disposable in various contexts.
7. **Love for Parents:** Cherish and value your parents, as they are the ones who offer unconditional love.

Earning :

1) **Family:** They are my greatest treasure and the center of my world.
2) **Blessings:** Grateful for the many blessings from those in my life.
3) **Friends:** Although few, my friends are invaluable gems.
4) **Impact:** The positive influence I have made on my students and colleagues.
5) **Spiritual Alignment:** Maintaining spiritual balance keeps me calm and motivated.
6) **Life Experiences:** Rich and diverse experiences that shape my journey.
7) **Confidence:** The self-assurance that drives my actions and decisions.

Expectation:

1) **Dignity:** Always maintain and preserve my dignity and self-respect.
2) **Better World:** Strive to make the world a better place for everyone.
3) **Productive Engagement:** Stay engaged and avoid idleness.
4) **Capability to Help:** Seek divine assistance to enhance my ability to help others.
5) **Environmental Awareness:** Foster a greater understanding of the importance of environmental preservation.

6) **Knowledge:** More time to read for increasing my knowledge
7) **Good Health:** I always remain healthy.

॥ ॐ ॥

Priyanka Sapraa

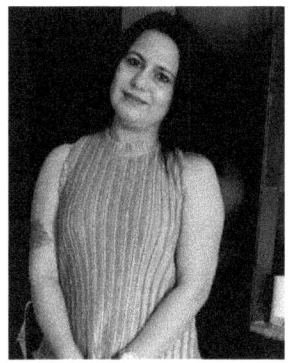

Author's Name	:	Priyanka Sapraa
Qualification	:	M.A. (Meditation & Yog) B.Ed., B.Lib., Diploma in Naturopathy
Current Profession	:	Occult Science Practitioner
Age	:	46 years
E-mail ID	:	priyankaramansapra@yahoo.com
City/ Country	:	**Gurugram, India**

Priyanka Sapraa is working as a Vastu Consultant & Numerologist. She's started her journey into occult science 23 years back, when she's joined her Master in Meditation & Yog from Jain Vishwa Bhartiya University, Ladnun, Rajasthan and a diploma course in yoga from Vivekananda Yog Anusandhan Samsthan, Bangalore.

Later in life she's learned that Yog is not only a physical exercise, but it's a greatest path to move towards your inner journey.

Later she's learned about Vastu and got to know more how a place can make an impact of anyone's Life through land energy and the 45 devtas are present in under a roof.

Learning new skills like Reiki, Nakshatra Jyotish, Medical Numerology, Mobile Numerology are the helping tools of her to bring more peace & harmony in anyone's Life.

Priyanka has the below LEEs of life :

Learning :

1. **Honesty** – This is the fastest way to prevent a mistake from turning into a failure.

2. **Confidence** – It opens up room for invention & discovery. Your success will be determined by your own confidence.

3. **Skills** – Try to upgrade your self with study & new skills.

4. **Positivity** – Being positivity of your life depends on the quality of your thoughts.

5. **Lend a helping hand** – Helping others is the secret sauce to a happy life.

6. **Self-respect** – Embrace the glorious mess that you are.

7. **Spirituality** – The intuitions builds you into a wonderful personality & take you to the right direction.

Earning :

1. **Strong Intuition** – I am able to trust more to existence and feel empowered.

2. **Optimum Health** – I love my body & it's my own responsibility to take care of it in a best way.

3. **Family** – The love & blessings from everyone in my ffamily 4. Dream house – My new home is the home of my happiest dream.

5. **Moral Values** – The moral values I have learned from my grand parents and now passing to my own child.

6. **Friends** – True friends who are always stand behind me & become a part of my family.

7. **Meditation** – it's a true love of your own company in an inner silence.

Expectation :

1. **Healthy Life** – I want to do Physical workout on daily basis till my last breath.

2. **Social Welfare** – I will be able work for social cause like educating street kids or women welfare.

3. **Care & Tenderness** – I wanna learn more about how to be more tenderness within myself to love & care others.

4. **Peace & harmony** – I expect to be able to achieve more peace and harmony with in myself.

5. **Success** – My definition of success is improving myself with each passing day.

6. **Practice Patience** – I have experienced that once patience conquered one can lead best life.

7. **Balanced Life** – Have more awareness in mind, love in the heart & righteousness in action to go ahead in the spiritual path.

|| ॐ ||

Prof. Sarojini Gupta Biddanda

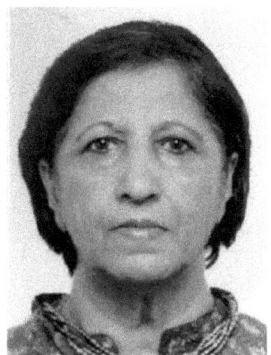

Author's Name	:	Prof. Sarojini Gupta Biddanda
Qualification	:	M.A. (English)
Current Profession	:	Retired Prof.
Age	:	71 years
E-mail ID	:	**sarojgupta369@yahoo.com**
City/ Country	:	**Coorg, Karnataka, India**

Prof. Sarojini Biddanda (Retd.) is an educationist with a distinguished career as a Professor of English and Principal of Kavery College (Degree) affiliated to the University of Mangalore. Her creative endeavors include writing and directing plays, choreographing theme based dances and composing songs. Her published poems are about nature, joys and sorrows of life. As a member of Lions Club, she plays an active role in the environmental and rural development projects undertaken by the club. She is a globe trotter with a passion for learning foreign languages. As a member of the Karnataka Kodava Sahithya Academy, she was instrumental in organizing folk music and dances during her tenure. She is also involved with prestigious literary and cultural associations.

There are many factors which contribute to make life wholesome and meaningful. We need the right direction to make it worth living. In this modern world people are preoccupied with the rat race and become oblivious of the things that are necessary for a purposeful life. They strive relentlessly to achieve material success at the cost of their well-being. Learning, earning and expectation are the three important aspects of life. Compiling ideas from successful and experienced people in an anthology will enable us to see life from different angles. Uniting writers from diverse walks of life on a single platform to share their perspectives on this topic **'Seven LEE of Life'** will help us broaden our horizons.

Learning :

1. **Knowledge:** Learning is a life long process of acquiring knowledge.
2. **School:** Early stage of learning is done at home and school where children learn to read, write and interact with others.
3. **Teaching:** Learning and teaching go together as teachers also learn while imparting knowledge to students.
4. **Growth:** Learning leads to personal growth and boosts one's creativity.
5. **Thinking:** Learning enhances our critical thinking and analyzing skills.
6. **Innovations:** Higher learning leads to orbit shifting innovations.
7. **Intellectual:** It fosters intellectual inclinations and shows us the path to rise above our ordinary selves.

Earning :

1. **Money:** In simple terms earning means money earned from a job or the profit from a business.
2. **Needs:** Earning money is essential to meet our day-to-day needs.
3. **End:** Earning money is a means to an end, but not an end to itself.
4. **Perspective:** Look at earning from a different perspective.
5. **Fame:** There are people who give a lot of importance to earning a good name and fame.
6. **Respect:** Earning respect and appreciation.
7. **Happiness:** Knowledge, unique experiences, happiness and peace of mind are more important than earning money.

Expectation :

1. **Life:** To lead a wholesome life.
2. **Education:** Education in the real sense of the word.
3. **Family:** Affectionate family and friends to fill my life with joy and meaning.
4. **Peace:** Peace of mind to live in harmony with the world.
5. **Service:** To render altruistic service to the society.
6. **Optimism:** Be optimistic and keep soaring.
7. **Unrealistic:** Avoid unrealistic expectations.

|| ॐ ||

Promila Devi Sutharsan Huidrom

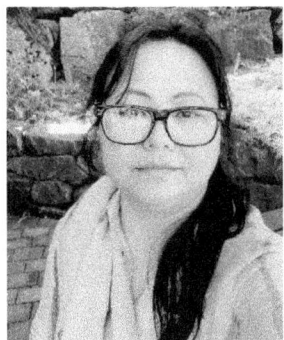

Author's Name	:	Promila Devi Sutharsan Huidrom
Qualification	:	Bachelor of Computer Science (B.C.S.), Diploma in Advanced Computing (C-DAC, Pune), MSc in Innovation and Entrepreneurship (Oslo, Norway)
Current Profession	:	Poet/ Author
Age	:	44 years
E-mail ID	:	**writerpromila@gmail.com**
City/ Country	:	**Jevnaker, Norway**

Promila Devi Sutharsan Huidrom/ Promila, being a modest Poetess, enjoys writing in Hindi and has been writing from a very young age. It has to be a path chosen formidably by her, quitting her Software and Business career. She has been residing in Norway for about 20 years now and settled and still write in Hindi and chose Hindi as the core language chosen for her writing, although her future books are coming in English and Norwegian too. She has won many Awards and accolades.

She is an active philanthropist and social reformer, who believe in giving the society back in the way, that which gave her an identity and life so beautiful.

Love life, live life and life is so beautiful.

Life is learning in every step, we gain, we lose and we learn. In each step whether we lose or gain we earn something which is the experience of life and with that the unaccomplished dreams could be made as a resolution and keep in our expectations. There is so much we all expect, what is relevant and how much time we have, we should manage to do whatever we can achieve. At the end of the day whether we fail or not, it's just a learning and adds as one step more towards success. No failure is a fail, it's just s path towards achievement. Live life to the fullest as if everyday is a celebration.

Learn to my best – Earn to Live and Expect to do more: That's life…

Learning :

1) **Life :** Life is a learning in every Phase

2) **Acceptance :** Acceptance is crucial as they are

3) **Duty :** Duties should be done at our best

4) **Light :** If there is bright light, there is darkness too, it's just a phase and brightness comes again

5) **Me-Time :** There should be always a "Me-Time" everyday even if it's little

6) **Read :** Read what you like to read everyday

7) **Write :** Write down your heart out and you will feel better

Earning :

1) **Children :** My Kids are my earning of life

2) **Words :** My Words which I prepared in the form of Book(s)

3) **Deeds :** My Deeds I did for needy

4) **Patience :** My Patience

5) **Will :** My Will

6) **Space :** My Space

7) **Virtues :** My Virtues

Expectation :

1) **Beyond :** Life beyond Life

2) **Help :** Help more to the needy

3) **Hobbies :** Could Pursue Painting, Sketching, Stiching and more

4) **Time :** Wish to have 3-4 hours more everyday

5) **Resource :** Mode of resource could be better and not currency

6) **Institution :** Dream to make an institution and beyond

7) **Live :** Wish the world understands better that "Live and Let Live" concept

|| ॐ ||

Punam Vishwkarma

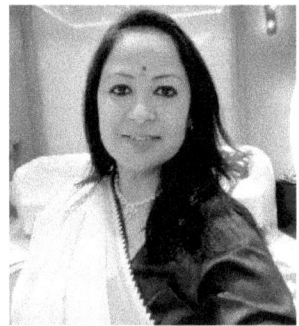

Author's Name	:	Punam Vishwkarma
Qualification	:	B.Sc., B.Ed., M.B.A. (HR)
Current Profession	:	Administration Head in School
Age	:	41 Years
E-mail ID	:	**punamvishwkarma055@gmail.com**
City/ Country	:	**Nagpur, India**

Punam Vishwkarma lives in tiger capital of India, Nagpur. She is a proud mother of two kids and wife of a handsome man. She is an Educationist, Guide and a Friend, these are her life blessings. She is a Tarot Card Reader and Numerologist. She helps people to decode the secrets of a successful life with numerology. She is a member of GLOAN, Global Alliance of Numerologists, which is a platform for Numerologist and Numerology seekers, all over the world to share quality information and conduct research in the field of Numerology.

Punam has the below LEEs of life :

Learning :

1. Numerology
2. Tarot Card Reading
3. Educationst
4. Technology
5. Financial Literacy
6. Car Driving

7. Gratitude Practicing

Earning :

1. Relationship, Career choice, & Personal development.
2. Confidence, Finance, Spirituality.
3. Professional growth, financially independent.
4. Self-development, increased job opportunities, confidence.
5. This helped me in gaining experience and confidence in making investment decisions.
6. Increased Independence, enjoyment, self-confidence.
7. Increased feeling of happiness, positivity, fulfillment & resilience into my life.

Expectation :

1. Giving more guidance on Career path and life purpose to people.
2. To help more people using tarot card, practice more spirituality.
3. Committed to help students learning and grow, promoting educational equity.
4. Continuous learning & updating skills to stay current with technological advancement.
5. Maintaining a long term perspective & understating different types of investments.
6. To buy an automatic new car.
7. To incorporate more gratitude into my daily life, I can try various practices that can help cultivate a mindset of thankfulness.

|| ॐ ||

Radhika Devgan

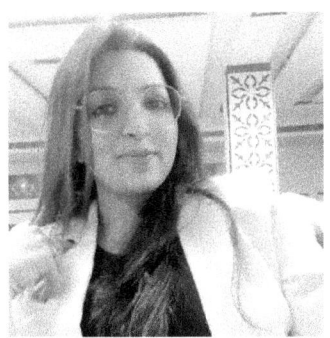

Author's Name	:	Radhika Devgan
Qualification	:	B.Sc. in Medical, M.C.A.
Current Profession	:	Immigration Consultant PTE, IELTS and OET Trainer, Las of Attraction Coach & NLP Trainer
Age	:	37 years
E-mail ID	:	86radhika@gmail.com
City/ Country	:	Punjab, India

Radhika Devgan is a well-established business woman. She started her career as a global language trainer in 2016 and continues in this role. Apart from her academic qualification in MCA, she pursued her interest in spiritualism and completed a Reiki Master Course in 2020-21. She is also a member of FICCIFLO Amritsar. Recently, she completed a basic level hypnotherapy course. As a science student, she had a great interest in science, particularly biological and chemical reactions in the body. Because of this, she is studying NLP and providing training to international students. Her aim is to educate everyone on how they can heal their own bodies and manifest all their dreams.

The **'Seven LEE of Life'** sheds light on the perspective of the human being toward life and the experiences encountered throughout the journey. Apart from this, he is the sculptor of his own life, and the tools he uses to shape it are patience, hard work, consistency, and a burning desire to create a perfect posture of life.

Learning :

1. **Education:** An education is a tool that can stay with us until our last breath.

2. **Me Time:** It's a time when we can spend time with the most beautiful creation of God: ourselves.
3. **Inner Peace:** Inner peace comes only with meditation. We need to listen to the inner voice, which is the actual voice of God.
4. **Positive Vibes:** Positive vibes can be created by adopting a positive attitude, such as meditation, positive thoughts, and positive words.
5. **Power of Words:** Words have tremendous power to change our lives. There are two types of words: what we speak and what we think.
6. **Power of Breath:** Breath is a universal energy. We can attract health, money, dreams, and achieve goals by consciously practicing deep breathing.
7. **Omnipresence of God:** God is within us. We just need to practice listening to the subtle voice of God. All creativity is within us.

Earning :

1. **Family Love:** The family love that reminds me every single moment that I am the wealthiest woman, although to earn this I had to pay in the form of money, patience, care, and attention.
2. **Positive Attitude:** It is just like a muscle that cannot be grown in a single day. We need to spend time and stay open in every moment, then we can get the identity of a positive person.
3. **Knowledge through Reading:** This is a real treasure that is gained through reading only. The answers to any situation are already given in books; we just need to create interest in them.
4. **Self-made Woman:** A woman is the only creature on this planet without whom the life of any organism is impossible. Everyone must explore the potential that is possible through awareness.
5. **Belief System:** A belief system can be developed by consistent thinking on a particular topic. This is the weapon to change our life by reprogramming our belief system.
6. **Spiritualism:** Its foundation is based upon calmness and focus. If we learn this perspective, life becomes very smooth.
7. **Health is Wealth:** We can enjoy our life only with a healthy body. The rest of the money is useless if our health is not working.

Expectation :

1. **Green Earth:** It's my goal to do something unique for Mother Earth by growing more trees.
2. **Sharing Knowledge:** If anyone has knowledge on a particular topic, we must share it, I want to share my knowledge of spiritualism worldwide.
3. **Build an NGO for the Needy:** There's no doubt we are blessed enough. God has made us complete. I want to build an NGO where everyone can avail benefits free of cost.

4. **Partnership with God:** "Tenth" is a term that started in Punjab, where we make a partnership with Almighty God. The profit of God is shared with other works of society. If everyone follows this concept, the majority of problems will disappear.

5. **Shelter for Strays:** Stray animals are also God's creations. We have to give them love by spending time with them and giving them food.

6. **God is One:** This intuition should be instilled in everyone's mind. We are human beings first, and God is omnipresent. There should be no discrimination. We should even share the knowledge of every religion with each other.

7. **Healing Centers:** In India, there is a need for healing centers like those in other foreign countries because every human being has the power to overcome chronic diseases. We need to work on the roots; a healthy life is the fruit.

|| ॐ ||

Raghunandan Chowdarapu

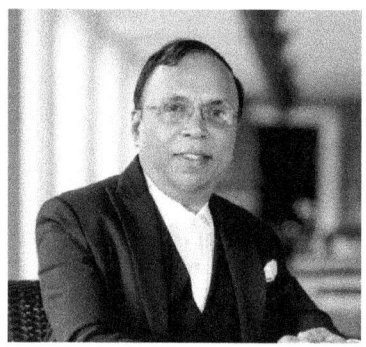

Author's Name	:	Raghunandan Chowdarapu (Raghu NC)
Qualification	:	B.A. – Triple Maths
Current Profession	:	Chairman of Magnifiq Group Companies
Age	:	63 years
E-mail ID	:	**ncraghu@gmail.com**
City/ Country	:	**Hyderabad, India**

Raghunandan Chowdarapu, with over four decades of experience in building businesses and fostering financial independence among entrepreneurs, has established himself as a seasoned expert in the industry.

He holds multiple Masters degrees in Mathematics and has undertaken numerous personal development courses, continually evolving his skills and knowledge.

As the founder of **Magnifiq Group Companies**, Raghunandan leads a conglomerate of successful enterprises. His unique expertise as a Master Practitioner in Graphology, combined with his profound knowledge in Astrology and Numerology, has empowered countless businesses to achieve remarkable growth. Raghunandan's holistic approach, blending scientific analysis and metaphysical insights, offers innovative strategies for personal and professional success. His dedication to financial awareness and entrepreneurial empowerment underscores his commitment to driving positive change in the business world.

Raghu's Seven LEE's are the cornerstones of his life

For Learning, I prioritize being trustworthy, always reliable and honest. Setting realistic goals and taking accountability for my actions are crucial. I keep my dreams alive, aspiring for a better future.

Effectiveness means maximizing resources and time. Bonding with family and friends is essential. Charity is a must, dedicating a fixed percentage of my income to those in need.

In Earning, I focus on giving affection and surrounding myself with love. I gather appreciation through kind actions and gain esteem through education and experiences. I maintain vigor with a healthy diet, yoga, and exercise. Tranquility is achieved through meditation and prayer. Dignity involves respecting others and fulfilling responsibilities. Prosperity is pursued with perseverance and wisdom, ensuring an abundant life.

My Expectations include accomplishment and success. Independence is key, allowing freedom for myself and others. Compassion guides me to forgive and move forward. Acceptance helps me trust in the divine plan. I strive for fairness, treating everyone equally. Clear dialogue and progress are constant goals.

Learning :

1) **Trust worthiness**: Being reliable & honest in all actions
2) **Realistic:** Setting practical & achievable goals
3) **Accountability:** Owning up to one's actions and their outcomes
4) **Dream:** A vision or aspiration for the future.
5) **Effectiveness:** Achieving desired results with the resources and time available.
6) **Bonding**: Maintaining excellent relationship with family & friends
7) **Charity**: Must give a fixed % of your income.

Earning :

1) **Affection**: Accumulate lots of love.
2) **Appreciation**: Gather blessings through kind actions.
3) **Esteem**: Gain greatness through education and experiences.
4) **Vigor**: Achieve good health through proper diet and exercise.
5) **Tranquility**: Attain a peaceful mind through meditation and prayer
6) **Dignity**: Earn respect by respecting others and fulfilling your responsibilities.
7) **Prosperity:** Achieve abundance through perseverance and wisdom.

Expectation :

1) **Accomplishment**: To succeed in life.
2) **Independence**: To live freely and allow others the same.
3) **Compassion**: To forgive and move on.
4) **Acceptance**: To trust in the divine plan.
5) **Fairness**: To treat everyone with equality.

6) **Dialogue**: To communicate clearly.
7) **Progress**: To grow and adapt to change

॥ ॐ ॥

Rahul Churi

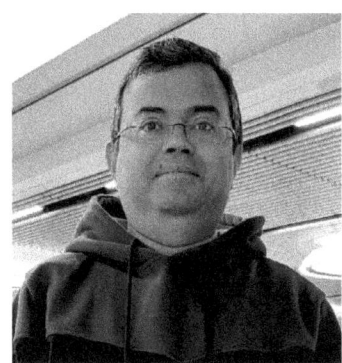

Author's Name	:	Rahul Churi
Qualification	:	B.Sc.
Current Profession	:	Assistant Professor in English
Age	:	50 years
E-mail ID	:	aashwa@yahoo.com
City/ Country	:	London, UK

Rahul Churi is an IT Consultant for 25+ years, belongs to Indian family. He loves to write and healthy discussion on the topic of relationship and society.

Rahul has the below LEEs of life :

Learning :

1) **Endless Learning:** Learning has no end no age.

2) **Adyhatmic Learning:** Understanding of Adhyatma is critical for happy life.

3) **Handling Prarabdha:** Learning is the only way a human can uplift the life from any Prarabdha.

4) **Calming Minds:** Learning will help calming the life energies.

5) **Amrut:** Vidya is equivalent to Amrut as a shloka explains and its true.

6) **Life Experiences:** Learning from life experiences is very important.

7) **Respect Teacher:** Anyone who teaches has to be respected as a guru in that field.

Earning :

1) **Purushartha:** Earning is "Purushartha" as per our Indic culture.
2) **Growth:** Growth is a wisdom from Indic culture that wealth creator is a Avatar.
3) **Home Wealth Creator:** Every home needs to have a central wealth creator.
4) **Wealth creation:** Wealth creation with detachment decides one's karma.
5) **Limitations:** Earning is dependent on the Prarabdha & Karmic combination.
6) **Charity:** "Yathashakti" based on one's capacity charity should be done.
7) **Pleasant Feeling:** Earnings should life of family as pleasant with values.

Expectation :

1) **Zero Expectations:** Any expectations will eventually create sadness.
2) **Expectations Source:** Source of expectations need understood so they don't come from last birth.
3) **Not Birth Right:** Any expectations however basic they may not be our birth right.
4) **Detachment:** Life is supposed to be lived with detachment to contain unruly expectation.
5) **Karmic Duties:** Expectations should only be seen in terms of Karmic duties.
6) **Non-Permanent:** Our expectations are not permanent and change with age and time.
7) **Ego:** Expectations associated with ego will eventually destroy the peace in one's life.

|| ॐ ||

Reva Sarangal

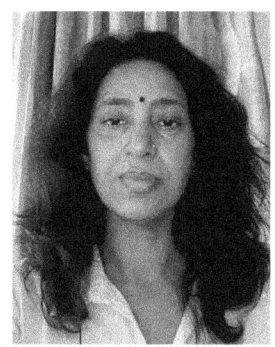

Author's Name	:	Reva Sarangal
Qualification	:	M.Sc. (Chemistry), M.Sc. (Ecology and Environment), B.Ed.
Current Profession	:	International Educator
Age	:	50 years
E-mail ID	:	**sarangalkakshi125@gmail.com**
City/ Country	:	**Mohali, India**

Reva Sarangal is an online International Educator with passion of teaching. Teaching gives her immense satisfaction. Even teaching for hours won't make her tired. She tries her best to motivate young minds to make their lives beautiful, happy and inspirational.

She believes –

IF YOUR PASSION BECOMES YOUR JOB THEN YOU ARE NEVER TIRED OF WORKING.

Reva believes that-make use of time as you cannot touch again the same water in the stream, so work hard to achieve your goals.

Life is too short; make it memorable, so that when looked back one should be contended and proud of it. Every individual has some role to play on this Earth and he does the same as destined by God. Once an individual leaves for ever, he/ she leaves a void, which never get filled. The lines of this song never appealed so much, but now every word means a lot and appears so true ;

Phool khilte hain, log miilte hain.

Phool khilte hain, log miilte hain,

Magar pattajhad men jo phool murajha jaate hain,

Vo bahaaron ke aane se khilte nahin…

Kuchh log ik roz jo bichhad jaate hain,

Vo hazaaron ke aane se milte nahin,

Umr bhar chaahe koi pukaara kare unakaa naam,

Vo phir nahin aate, vo phir nahin aate…

We are here on Earth for some cause. God has blessed us with unique opportunities and experiences. Everything that happens in life is because of some reason. It has God's plan. We should take life with a motive to nake it worth living so that we shouldn't regret later. Keep faith in HIS plan and do the right. At the end of the day just check what all you did right from the morning till going to bed. If you are not sorry for anything you have done through out the day means you made through best of it.

Live a life which is inspirational to other and be thankful to GOD that you are here.

Reva has the below LEEs of life :

Learning :

1. Always learn from mistakes.
2. Love everyone.
3. Respect others.
4. Forget and forgive.
5. Add something everyday to your knowledge
6. Don't burden others.
7. Try to solve your problems on your own.

Earning :

1. Respect from my students and friends.
2. Faith of my friends and family.
3. Contentment from life.
4. Trust of my loved ones.
5. Humility, I am humble to everyone.
6. Knowledge from life and academics.
7. God's faith to believe in him.

Expectation :

1. Everyone shuld be truthful.
2. Life should be full of happiness.

3. Feeling of gratitude should be there.
4. Be contended with what i have.
5. My actions and words shouldn't hurt others.
6. Life shuld not be harsh.
7. Love, care and respect.

॥ ॐ ॥

Rita Sehgal

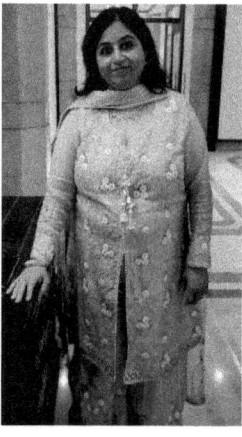

Author's Name	:	Rita Sehgal
Qualification	:	Graduate
Current Profession	:	Professional Vastu Consultant, Certified Numerologist Astrologer, Tarot Card Reader, Dowsing Expert, Certified Published Author, The Owner of Lions Den lounge
Age	:	54 years
E-mail ID	:	**ritasehgal18.rs@gmail.com**
City/ Country	:	**Kolkata, India**

Rita Sehgal is here to serve her soul mission of helping and transforming lives through her expertise in occult science and intuition. She has over seven years of experience in this field and has consulted clients globally, offering them profound knowledge and insights.

Life has been a great teacher, offering me lessons that continue to guide my journey. One of the most important lessons that I have learned is the value of patience. Growth does not happen overnight, it often comes from overcoming difficulties and discomforts. Caring for your health is the most valuable investment we can make. We should try to respect others opinions and understand their point of view only then we can truly value our relationship. Time has a remarkable ability to heal, while failures rather than being my setbacks, have been my most effective teachers showing me what does not work and helping me discover what does. Embracing change is essential because nothing in life stays the same. Learning to adopt to situations has made my journey easy and have been key to my personal growth. Spirituality has also become a significant part of my life providing me with a deeper sense of meaning and connection to something beyond myself. This spiritual foundation gives me peace and helps me navigate life challenges with greater clarity. Always being grateful for all the blessings in my life has kept me grounded. Gratitude is a must. Wisdom has been one of the greatest rewards which I have acquired through years of learning and self-reflection. Inner peace have become priceless asset which helped me to keep calm when faced with life challenges. I have built a lot of confidence by trusting in myself. Throughout life I have gained a lot of valuable experiences and respect. We should always strive to find ways to make a positive impact on the lives of those around us.

Learning :

1. Patience
2. Embrace Change
3. Value Relationship
4. Health is Wealth
5. Failures are the stepping stones to success
6. Gratitude brings Peace
7. Time Heals

Earning :

1. Wisdom from Experience
2. Love from Giving
3. Strength from Struggle
4. Peace from Forgiveness
5. Self respect
6. Trust
7. Spirituality

Expectation :

1. Seek Balance in All Things
2. Cherish The Simple Moments
3. Be open to Learning in Every Stage
4. Aspire for Growth Not Perfection
5. Trust That Unseen Forces Guide Your Journey
6. Spiritual Enlightenment
7. Positive Impact on People's Lives

|| ॐ ||

Rohan Jain

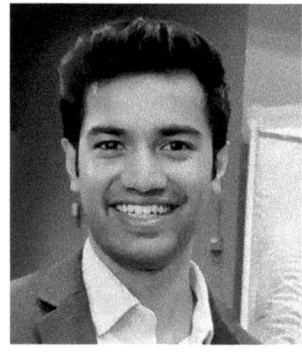

Author's Name	:	Rohan Jain
Qualification	:	BBA, MBA
Current Profession	:	Business
Age	:	26 Years
E-mail ID	:	rohan@texcarp.com
City/ Country	:	Pune, India

Rohan Jain is based in Pune and lives in a close-knit family with his wife, parents and grandparents. A management graduate with a specialization in marketing, he joined his family business in 2019 after completing his studies. He aspires to build on the foundation that his father has set up and diversify the business into new verticals. To reinforce this goal, he has also completed his masters in family managed business. A strong believer in work life balance, he loves to spend his free time with his family, reading books and playing table tennis.

I believe that this topic effectively captures the broad pillars that constitute an individual's life. No matter what we are doing in life, we are more often than not either learning something, taking actions through which we earn something and we expect certain outcomes based on those actions.

A divine number, 108 co-authors sharing their personal learning, earning and expectation will provide a beautiful and interesting snapshot of how perspectives change amongst people who are in different stages in life and who come from various backgrounds.

Learning :

1) **Values:** My parents have instilled values in me that guide me in making key decisions in life

2) **Education in Management:** Having done my graduation and post-graduation in management has enabled me to ably contribute in my business

3) **Value of Time:** I have learned to always be punctual, value my own time and that of others too

4) **Health is Priority:** A person can have everything yet enjoy nothing if they are plagued by health issues. Hence for me maintaining good health is the most important in life.

5) **Habits:** Your habits can make or break your life so its always important to hold on to good ones and let go of the bad ones

6) **Always think Positive:** I have learned that no matter how difficult life may seem at times, if you try to see the positive side of things you can surmount any challenge.

7) **Gratitude is the Key:** Always be thankful for everything that you have and never fail to thank the people around you.

Earning :

1) **Unending love and support:** I receive an immense amount of love and support from my parents and wife.

2) **Valuable friendships:** I have just a few but very close friends whom I can always count on.

3) **Financial stability:** I am glad that I earn a stable income and have enough investments to support my and my family's needs and for things that I enjoy

4) **Respect of my peers:** I am fortunate to be respected by my family, friends and colleagues

5) **A Fulfilling career:** I am a part of my family business, and this has provided me with opportunities to interact with international organisations and practically implement my academic knowledge

6) **Contentment:** I am overall content with what I have in life. That doesn't imply that I don't have any aspirations, but I don't feel like anything is missing

7) **Robust self-confidence:** My academic background and international exposure through our business has greatly built up my self confidence and self esteem

Expectation :

1) **Continued personal growth:** I wish to continue to gain opportunities to grow my knowledge and further refine my skills

2) **Opportunities to contribute towards society:** I want to be given avenues through which I can contribute more towards society and for the betterment of people's lives

3) **Further success in business:** I would like to put more efforts into business and continue to grow it year on year

4) **Work-life balance:** I already have a good work life balance and would like to maintain it through active efforts and good structuring of my time

5) **Maintenance of my well-being:** I wish to be able to devote enough time and energy towards maintaining my physical and mental well-being

6) **Challenging situations:** I would also like to experience challenging situations now and then which would make me stronger and give me a chance to prove myself

7) **Opportunity for creativity:** I would like opportunities to create something entirely new using my creativity, both in the personal as well as professional space.

|| ॐ ||

Rohet B Kummbar

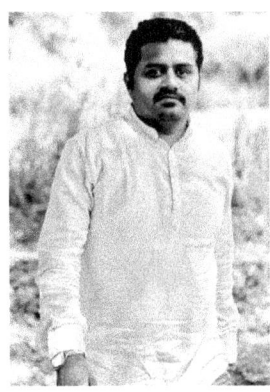

Author's Name	:	Rohet B Kummbar
Qualification	:	B.Tech. (Chemical)
Current Profession	:	Consultant and Organiser
Age	:	34 years
E-mail ID	:	**rohitkumbhar31@gmail.com**
City/ Country	:	**Kolhapur, Maharashtra, India**

Rohet B Kummbar studied B. Tech in Chemical and worked as a Production Engineer for 2 years. Since he did not like a bonded job, he associated himself with network marketing to start his own business. Due to his interest in studying spirituality, he participated in meditation camps and satsangs. For the past 4 years, he has established an educational and consultation academy by the name of Sadhna Healing Hub, where through his experience many people are getting trained in occult sciences and spirituality. He is a Professional Numerologist and Vastu Consultant; due to his interest in occult sciences, he remains engaged in new research.

'**Seven LEE**' means Learning, Earning & Expectation, these are interconnected. According to my experience, these three aspects have a very important contribution in our life. Like whatever option or resolution or goal we have in our life, that is the thing around us that is attractive and you start moving forward with that only.

Seven is a number that is connected with existence and is a number connected with many dimensions of our life. If a person has to move forward on the path of spiritual advancement through the truth cycle of energy, then this number is also important from the spiritual point of view.

So life is a journey and every person has different understanding and experience in life. So when we are in any situation, we need to focus on what life is teaching us. This one thing will make you develop as a conscious and mature person towards life.

Learning :

1. **Keep the body pure and healthy:** If you are healthy and fit, you can find joy and goals in life.
2. **Emotional development and balance:** Purity of your emotions is essential for building relationships and feelings of belongingness.
3. **Understand your own mind:** This understanding is useful in the development of our mental abilities and in worldly life.
4. **Manage relationships:** Sweetness, love and a feeling of belongingness in relationships make good relationships.
5. **Acceptance towards life:** Accepting whatever is happening in life deepens our awareness and understanding.
6. **Practice gratitude:** Having acceptance towards life begins the practice of gratitude in our life.
7. **Be curious for self-knowledge:** The curiosity to seek knowledge and soul knowledge helps you to develop spiritually.

Earning :

1. **Wisdom, Knowledge and Skills:** Wisdom comes from practice while knowledge and skills can be acquired through education.
2. **Career:** It is important to achieve financial freedom and professional goals.
3. **Patience:** Patience is important in our changing circumstances, it helps to face challenges.
4. **Blessings & Grace:** Connecting with sacred energy gives a positive impact and a peaceful experience in our life work.
5. **Take responsibility:** Whatever responsibility you have, make it a part of your life and try to handle it.
6. **Move forward with determination:** Determination is the key to fulfilling every purpose of life.
7. **Achievements:** Success is not just defined as financial growth, but it means having a positive impact in the lives of others and connecting with each other in a soulful way.

Expectation :

1. **Personal Growth:** Growing as a person through experiences motivates us.
2. **Security:** Feeling emotionally, physically, financially and mentally safe is something everyone desires.
3. **Respect:** Respect includes having your ideas respected. Your efforts and achievements are valued by those around you.

4. **Balance:** It is important to balance your inner dimensions and manage your time and energy effectively.

5. **Purpose in Life:** A sense of purpose makes life positively fulfilling and fulfillment

6. **Positive Relationships:** Positive relationships with family, friends and close ones enrich our lives. These relationships provide emotional support and a sense of belonging.

7. **Spiritual Growth:** Spiritual growth increases the strength of our soul. Oneness with a sacred power and spiritual growth leads to inner peace and an ability to know and explore the world around us.

॥ ॐ ॥

Romi Maakan

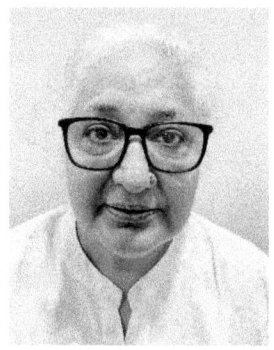

Author's Name	:	Romi Maakan
Qualification	:	Graduate
Current Profession	:	Law of Attraction Coach and Healer
Age	:	62+ years
E-mail ID	:	**contact.thesoulradiance@gmail.com**
City/ Country	:	**New Delhi, India**

Romi Maakan is a renowned Gratitude and Law of Attraction coach with over 25 years of experience in helping people transform their lives through healing practices and manifestation techniques. She holds multiple certifications including Ho'Oponopono Healing, Chakra healing, NLP and life coaching.

She's the founder and CEO of The Soul Radiance, an organization dedicated to holistic healing and self-empowerment. Her 30-day gratitude challenges and workshops have gone global and set the agenda for framing positive mental well-being and personal growth. Passionate to develop self-love, resilience, and compassion, Romi further inspires people to have gratitude and lead richly fulfilling lives.

Empowering Your Path Through Life's Core Principles

Learning :

1. **L - Listen :** I am proud to say my learning was only possible because I became a good listener. It opened my mind and made me willing to absorb teachings like a sponge. I learned from my miseries.

2. **E - Explore :** When I became a good listener, I explored and shared with future generations and all the seekers to follow, helping them live a life of abundance.

3. **A - Acquire :** All the learning my miserable life pushed me to acquire, made me a sponge for life lessons that travel from soul to soul. Wow!

4. **R - Reflect :** Now my learning allows me to reflect on the actions I took in miserable times and how they created miracles. Wow! I now teach this passionately, and all the seekers come to me seeking solutions. No wonder together, we are all creating miracles.

5. **N – Nurture :** I nurtured my soul practically by implementing the guidance of the universe, and miracles were created.

6. **I - Integrate :** It mesmerizes me how integration occurred from all my learnings, creating a life formula for miracles that even my generations have started following.

7. **N - Non-negotiable :** Honestly speaking, learning is a non-negotiable tool that has assured me massive success in every area of my life, be it health, relationships, career, or money.

   G – Gratitude !!!

Earning :

1. **E - Earning :** My learning is that the real earnings of life are the assets that can travel with your soul through lifetimes.

2. **A - Achieve :** My true life learnings made me achieve all the earnings that helped me attain real balance between health, wealth, wisdom, and time freedom. Wow, what more could I achieve!

3. **R – Rewards :** Real rewards are true earnings, and when you leave them as a legacy for future generations, even they are secured. Universe, thank you, thank you, thank you for such big rewards.

4. **N - Navigate :** The miseries of my life navigated me toward earnings, and learning played a vital role in transforming my miseries into miracles.

5. **I – Invest :** Today, I wonder how, during the most miserable period of my life, the moment I started investing in my learning, it became the perfect tool for divine earnings that created a miraculous life for me. Universe, thank you, thank you, thank you.

6. **N – Nurturing :** All my life's lessons are nurturing my soul and the souls of seekers to live a blessed life, even in this incarnation. What a blessed souls tribe we are now! Universe, thank you, thank you, thank you.

7. **G - Gratitude :** Trust me, gratitude has been the only tool in my life that turned all mysteries into miracles. And now, it is available to the whole of humanity. Universe, thank you, thank you, thank you for making me such a grateful soul.

Expectation :

1. **E – Evaluate :** Each day, in every way, evaluating each step and decision correctly can create miraculous learnings and earnings within me. Wow, what an evaluation!

2. **X – Explore :** My miseries drove me to explore different methods and, at times, to reevaluate myself as a coach. The moment I explored this, it gave me a full sense of purpose and filled my life with meaning.

3. **P - Prioritize :** When life reached rock bottom again during the pandemic, the universe prioritized coaching for me. Now, my passion brings miracles, not just to my life but also to the lives of all the souls reaching me, who have become magnets for miracle.

4. **E - Empower :** Wow, the sole purpose of my life now is to empower seekers who are looking for unlimited miracles. My purpose is to empower souls. Universe, thank you, thank you, thank you.

5. **T - Thrive :** The more I am committed to my mission and vision, the more my passion drives me. I am attracting exponential growth with every breath.

6. **I - Integrate :** It's miraculous to see how integrating Learning, Earning, and Expectations has made me thrive. These elements have given me this miraculous life, and I cherish the rewards with every breath.

7. **O - Optimize :** Optimizing my coaching journey is truly the path the universe started for me, and I am now rocking on my divine path, fulfilling all my material responsibilities. Universe, thank you, thank you, thank you for showing me the right path.

|| ॐ ||

Sadhana Athinamilagi

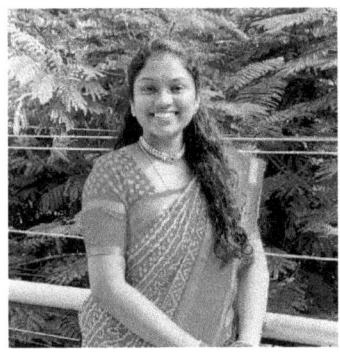

Author's Name	:	Sadhana Athinamilagi
Qualification	:	B.E Instrumentation Engineering
Current Profession	:	Lead Software Engineering
Age	:	28 years
E-mail ID	:	sadhanaathi77@gmail.com
City/ Country	:	Trichy, India

Sadhana Athinamilagi, an Engineering Graduate turned Data Engineer, is a passionate advocate for lifelong learning and personal development. Inspired by the transformative power of literature, she embarked on a journey to establish herself as a writer with the goal of making a meaningful impact on people's lives. What sets her apart is her unique approach to exploring these topics, continuously evolving as she delves deeper into her craft.

Beyond her writing endeavors, Sadhana is also an avid explorer of diverse interests like Art and Craft. She finds joy in delving into Yoga and practising meditation. As a mother, Sadhana aspires to be a source of inspiration for her daughter, imparting not only wisdom gained from professional and personal experiences but also a sense of wonder and curiosity about the world.

The **'Seven LEE's of Life'** — Learning, Earning and Expectation, offer a blueprint for fulfilling existence;

Learning emphasizes continuous personal growth and the acquisition of knowledge, essential for expanding our horizons and evolving as individuals.

Earning encompasses not just financial prosperity but also the accumulation of meaningful experiences, valuable relationships, and skills that enrich our journey.

Expectation drives us forward by nurturing aspirations and guiding our efforts towards achieving personal and professional goals, instilling a sense of purpose and direction in life. These principles collectively shape a holistic approach to living, encouraging us to embrace curiosity, ambition and a proactive mindset.

By integrating these elements, individuals can cultivate a balanced and meaningful life, characterized by continuous learning, meaningful contributions and a sense of fulfilment.

Learning :

1. Learn from exploration and failures to grow.
2. Follow your passion and do what you love.
3. Embrace impermanence and cherish moments.
4. Cultivate gratitude and find happiness in simplicity.
5. Set ambitious goals and strive for achievement.
6. Socialize and influence meaningful connections.
7. Prioritize your health for a balanced life.

Earning :

1. **Knowledge:** Continuous learning and intellectual growth.
2. **Experience:** Accumulation of life lessons and practical skills.
3. **Connections:** Building a network of valuable and supportive relationships.
4. **Freedom:** Ability to make choices and live authentically.
5. **Inner Peace:** Deepening your connection with your spirituality and inner self.
6. **Environmental Care:** Contributing to the sustainability and health of our planet.
7. **Legacy:** Making a positive impact that lasts beyond one's lifetime.

Expectation :

1. **Happiness:** Discover joy in every moment, whether significant or small.
2. **Love:** Cultivate empathy and kindness to nurture deep connections.
3. **Health:** Maintain well-being through physical, mental, and emotional care.
4. **Success:** Achieve personal and professional goals through persistence and development.
5. **Purpose:** Seek meaning and direction in life's journey.
6. **Balance:** Harmonize work, relationships, and self-care for overall wellness.
7. **Spirituality:** Explore beliefs for inner peace and connection.

|| ॐ ||

Sapna Gaurav Gupta

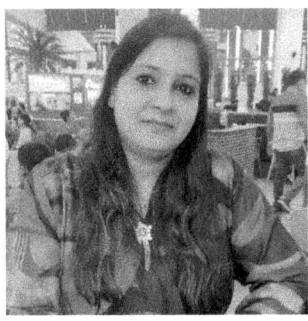

Author's Name	:	Sapna Gaurav Gupta
Qualification	:	B.Com.
Current Profession	:	Teacher, Counselor and Coach
Age	:	47 years
E-mail ID	:	**sgdream22@gmail.com**
City/ Country	:	**Mumbai, India**

Mrs. Sapna Gupta is a Cheerful and Passionate Educator with an impressive 25 years of experience in teaching and guiding students. Beyond conventional teaching, she has excelled as a mentor, helping students improve their handwriting skills as an expert graphologist, thus playing a pivotal role in grooming their personalities and boosting their confidence.

In addition to her expertise in graphology, Mrs. Gupta is a professional numerologist, logo analyst and designer, wristwatch analyst, and drawing analyst. These diverse skills have allowed her to provide comprehensive guidance and support, enriching the lives of thousands of individuals. Her profound knowledge in these areas has enabled her to add tremendous value to people's lives, helping them achieve personal growth and success.

Mrs. Gupta's influence extends beyond her professional life. She is also an avid traveller who finds joy in exploring new places and immersing herself in the diverse cultures and traditions of each destination. Through her extensive experience, diverse skills, and personal interests, Mrs. Sapna Gupta continues to inspire and positively impact the lives of many, leaving a lasting impression in the field of education and personal development.

Life is a roller coaster, full of ups and downs. As we navigate these peaks and valleys, we gain valuable insights, earn achievements and develop fresh aspirations. A smooth pathway will make our life monotonous and unfulfilling. More the challenges and hardships we face deeper we go with our learnings and experiences. It's only the challenges of life that enables us to create new opportunities and hence unearth our true potentials. This understanding shifts us to a higher level of Self-awareness and personal growth. We become more confident to set higher goals and continue to grow. This leads us to Success (our higher self).

Learning :

1) Things will fall for you at the right time and right pace – always stay Positive.

2) Set your Goals. Be consistent towards it.

3) Live Your Dreams, no one will live for you.

4) There is no age bar to Learning – keep learning as the world keeps changing.

5) Share your learnings – sharing makes you Wiser.

6) Always become a Giver, to be an Achiever.

7) Certain situations are not in our control. Live up to the Almighty God.

Earning :

1) Embarking on my journey as a Graphologist, I experienced profound spiritual growth that led to a transformational phase. I express my deepest gratitude to all my GURUS for their guidance and wisdom.

2) Inner calmness and happiness enriched my Relationships.

3) Mentorship helped me earn Respect and Love from my students. Which is my true reward, far beyond any material gain.

4) I live a life free of regrets. Unburdened by grudges.

5) I have no enemies, just few and true and cherished FRIENDS.

6) Realisation of my goals led to Self-satisfaction, affirming my journey and efforts.

7) Balance of personal and professional life has been a key of my well-being.

Expectation :

1) To bring positive difference in the lives of people who connect with me in the journey of life, guiding them toward a growth and fulfilment.

2) To confront and conquer my own inner fears.

3) Embracing self-care to lead a balanced life where wellness is my core focus.

4) To contribute positively to the underprivileged to create a positive change in the society.

5) A desire to explore the world drives me crazy for a family world tour.

6) I envision a peaceful retirement, amidst the beauty of nature, enjoying the finest companionship with my partner.

7) Cultivating inner peace by meditation.

॥ ॐ ॥

Sharlet Seraphim

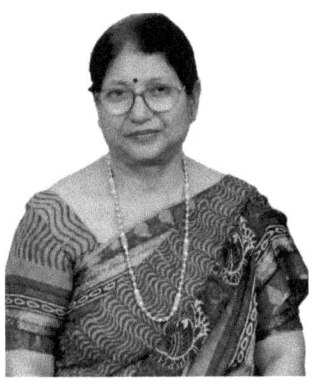

Author's Name	:	Sharlet Seraphim
Qualification	:	M.A, B.Ed.
Current Profession	:	Retired Teacher
Age	:	68 years
E-mail ID	:	**sharlet.seraphim@gmail.com**
City/ Country	:	**Gurgaon, India**

Sharlet Seraphim is a retired educationist. She has taught humanities to senior secondary students in Bihar Government for 33 years impacting lives of around 5000 students during her professional journey. She specializes in national and international history of modern era. She has keen interest in current affairs and is an avid reader. She has two daughters and currently lives in Gurgaon. As a retired professional she is currently pursuing her passion of cooking, baking, travelling and spending time with grandchildren.

Sharlet Seraphim has the below LEEs of life :

Learning :

1. **Sharing:** By sharing love and sorrow, we get strength to survive in this world.
2. **Family:** Each family has its own culture and traditions which gives different experiences.
3. **Adjustment**: Adjustment plays key role in family and society.
4. **Inner Strength**: A strong mind and a strong personality is always built and nurtured in a strong family background.
5. **Happiness and Fulfilment:** Life is full of demands, uncertainties and struggle but the family is the safe nest which gives us happiness and fulfilment.

6. **Support:** No matter, how much you earn or how much you lose, family is something which is always on your back supporting you.

7. **Enjoyment:** Family is a unit where there is a complete enjoyment with friends across different age groups in the form of your spouse, children, parents and in-laws who usually have fun despite their differences and some moments of anger, every now and then. People forget their fights and slowly learn to ignore and keep coming back to each other.

Earning :

1. **Impact:** The happiness gained have given a totality to my life experiences.

2. **Friends:** Friends that I have made along with family members do have a great importance in life.

3. **Values:** The values of humanity that I learnt and passed on to my children are precious to me.

4. **Experience:** The different stages of life has given me experiences that has made me what I am today, strong and independent.

5. **Fruitful Result:** Whatever hardship came in life, I embraced it as somehow, it has given me fruitful results later and made my soul happy.

6. **Wisdom:** Wisdom is a gift by birth that can only be acquired to an extent and results to amazing outcomes.

7. **Tolerance:** Family always imparts a lesson of tolerance, resulting in calm and peaceful character.

Expectation :

1. **Children's Well Being:** I wish my children and grandchildren are always happy and become socially responsible and wise citizens of the world having some unique impact within their capacity.

2. **Old Age:** Enjoy and cherish the rest of the time on earth peacefully and meaningfully and spend memorable time with my children.

3. **Contribute to Society:** Leverage platforms to contribute to society with my experiences and skills.

4. **Like Minded Companionship:** Be able to spend time with like-minded, spiritually evolved people.

5. **Spread Love:** To be able to spread love specially with those in need and have no one around.

6. **Health:** Lead a healthy life so that I can enjoy the blessings of the world.

7. **Family:** Family continues to be my pillar and I look forward to be surrounded by them and enjoy their love.

|| ॐ ||

Sheetal Pratik

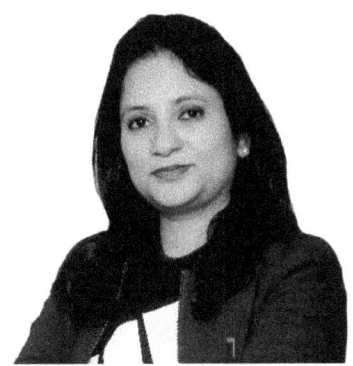

Author's Name	:	Sheetal Pratik
Qualification	:	BE (Electronics and Communication) BIT MESRA MBA (Systems) – IMT Ghaziabad
Current Profession	:	Director Engineering – Data and Analytics
Age	:	44 years
E-mail ID	:	**Shietal.paratik@gmail.com**
City/ Country	:	**Gurgaon, India**

Sheetal Pratik is a Data Leader, who has enabled organizations to deliver business values from data. With around 20+ years of experience in data related technologies at large organizations and start-ups, she has held various roles architecting and delivering data platforms across companies such as Oracle, Colt, NaviSite, Syntel, Mphasis, Reliance Jio Payments Bank, Saxo Bank and Adidas.

Currently she is working as Director Data Engineering, Data and Analytics at NatWest.

She holds a B.E. degree with distinction, from BIT Mesra in Electronics and Communication and is also a postgraduate in Business Administration from IMT Ghaziabad.

She has authored two research papers on data mesh and her paper on "Data Mesh Adoption: a Multi-case and Multi-method Readiness Approach" has won the Best Overall Paper award in December 2023, at EMCIS (European, Mediterranean and Middle Eastern Conference on Information Systems) The British University in Dubai.

She was interviewed for her work in 2022 by Harvard Business review on 'Creating Business Value with Data Mesh' for rolling out one of the early federated data governance platform.

In 2022, she received Indian Achievers Award 2022 by Indian Achievers Forum.

Sheetal Pratik has the below LEEs of life :

Learning :

1. **Explore** – Be open to explore what is there in life, as it might not go exactly as you plan.
2. **Acceptance** – Change what you can, accept what you cannot and ignore everything else as we have chosen our life and journey.
3. **Forgiveness** – Keep your heart and head light by making it free of any grudges.
4. **Purpose** – Do find your purpose of life and live for it every day.
5. **Happiness** – Decide to be happy no matter what, happiness is a decision and will not come from others.
6. **Love** – Love yourself unconditionally.
7. **Compromise** – Compromises made for your loved ones is not a sacrifice, it's a choice for your happiness.

Earning :

1. **Health** – My body is a temple for my soul and keeping it healthy is important so that my soul to be happy.
2. **Family** – My loved ones are my true assets and earning their love is a jewel.
3. **Impact** – The difference I have been able to make in others life, helped make people's career, offered help when people needed and thus turned around their future.
4. **Friends** – Cherishing and keeping friends who have stood through times.
5. **Values** – Values that I have been able to cultivate in me and pass on to my children.
6. **Experiences and Memories** – The beautiful moments with family, friends, pride, love and accomplishments are my true asset.
7. **Wisdom and Knowledge** – Knowledge collected in life via trainings, meeting people, parenting and working is my pillar for leading life beyond.

Expectation :

1. **Fulfillment and Happiness** – I want to find fulfillment by meeting my purpose of life to evolve into my higher self and keeping everyone around me happy.
2. **Good Settlement of my Children** – The most important dream for me is to see my children become good human beings and make a positive impact to the society.
3. **Health** – I expect myself and my family to be healthy and fit and continue to enjoy the gifts of life.
4. **Respect** – I expect to continue making impact on lives through my life and my work and thus earn respect and honor for myself and my family.

5. **Love and Peace** – Love, peace and harmony is essential for a happy life, and I continuously strive for the same in my family and surroundings and choose to walk away otherwise.

6. **Personal growth and development** – I strive for continuous growth and development both intellectually and emotionally by learning new skills, gain wisdom though experiences, and evolving as a person over time.

7. **Success** – Define my own success definition and continuous work towards that success and purpose of life.

|| ॐ ||

Shelaj Kant

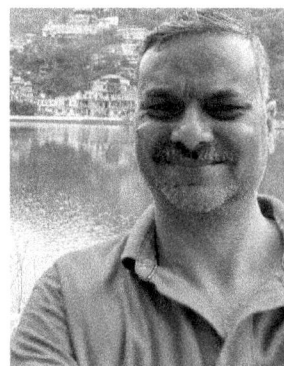

Author's Name	:	Shelaj Kant
Qualification	:	M.Sc. (Chemistry), B.Ed. Diploma in Naturopathy and yoga
Current Profession	:	PGT Chemistry
Age	:	47 years
E-mail ID	:	**Shelajssis@gmail.com**
City/ Country	:	**Dharamsala, India**

Shelaj Kant is Post Graduate Teacher in Chemistry. He has done his Master Degrees in Chemistry with speciation in Organic Chemistry. Worked more than 20 years as PGT Chemistry in reputed schools in India and UAE

He has completed three years Diploma in Naturopathy and Yoga.

Shelaj Kant`s current area of focus is Trigonum Numerology and is exploring extensive reading of books and research papers.

He loves to spend his leisure reading, cooking and exploring mountains.

'Seven LEE of Life' refers to fundamental values, principles that give life meaning and direction. My understanding of this topic:

Before we embark on journey of life, we must settle down on one important issue that is what do I want out of life and start working in that direction. Once I decided what I want from my life I should not stop till the cup is full. We have to move on we have to struggle and we have to try hard, we have to be disciplined in life till goal is achieved and that is the end of life. What we want out of life is peace, that will give us happiness and joy. that will give us fulfilment in life. It can not be a borrowed object; it has to be your own individual goal. If we set a very high goal and if we keep very high goal and we keep slugging we will repent on last day of life. Our goal in life must be SMART.

Goal should be clear concise and well defined

Goal should have a way to track progress

Goal should not be impractical

Goal should align with our philosophy of life and it must have some timeline for completion

Learning :

1. **Help:** Activity of contributing towards family, society and at large nation
2. **Bliss:** Perfect happiness
3. **Adaptibility:** survival in all circumstances
4. **Gratitude:** Art of appreciation of others good work
5. **Dissolve:** mix-up without losing your identity
6. **Liberate:** free from ego and anger
7. **Discipline and Determination:** Discipline propels us forward in life, determination teach us never give up

Earning :

1. **Discipline:** Discipline is most precious earning, shaping our character
2. **Adaptibility:** Overcome obstacles in life and stay focused
3. **Mindfulness:** Mindfulness is gift of God to cultivate inner piece
4. **Gratitude:** Art of appreciation is ultimate wealth
5. **Health:** Health is wealth
6. **Earning:** Purpose of Life
7. **Satisfaction:** reward of life

Expectation :

1. **Discipline:** Life's biggest expectations is self-discipline
2. **Adaptibility:** life expects us to adjust and adapt to its unpredictable nature.
3. **Mindfulness:** live life in present moment
4. **Satisfaction:** life's biggest ask is to live satisfied life
5. **Self-sufficient:** life expects us to be self-sufficient and independent
6. **Peace:** Mental peace around
7. **Growth:** Overall growth in life

|| ॐ ||

Shelly Arora

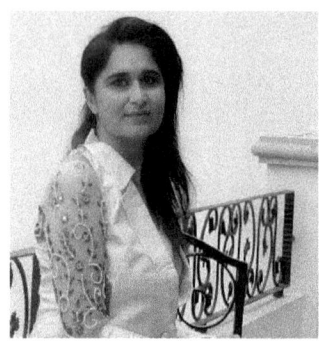

Author's Name	:	Shelly Arora
Qualification	:	Graduate
Current Profession	:	Consultant and Counselor in Occult Science
Age	:	42 years
E-mail ID	:	**anantadrishtishelly@gmail.com**
City/ Country	:	**Amritsar, India**

Shelly Arora is a co-founder of Anantadrishti Infinity Eye of Shiv. For over five years, she has dedicated herself to the world of occult practices. Her expertise spans a variety of disciplines, including healing, numerology, tarot card reading, rune reading, angel therapy, Akashic reading and glass ball gazing. As an award-winning rune reader, she has been recognized for her deep understanding and application of ancient wisdom. Shelly's work as an NLP coach and life consultant allows to guide individuals toward their true potential, helping them overcome obstacles and achieve their personal and professional goals. At Anantadrishti Infinity Eye of Shiv, aim to provide holistic guidance and support, empowering the clients with the knowledge and tools they need to lead fulfilling lives.

The **"Seven LEE of Life"** represents Physical, Emotional, Mental, Spiritual, Energetic, Social and Environmental levels.

Environmental Level: This involves our relationship with nature and the planet. It's about sustainability, harmony with the environment and ecological consciousness.

Learning :

1. **Physical:** Understand and care for your body and health

2. **Emotional:** Recognize and manage your emotions effectively
3. **Mental:** Develop your intellect and mindset
4. **Spiritual:** Connect with your inner self and the divine.
5. **Energetic:** Balance and harness your energy
6. **Social:** Build meaningful relationships and community bonds
7. **Environmental:** Foster a sustainable and harmonious relationship with nature.

Earning :

1. **Learning:** Continuously acquire new skills and knowledge to increase your earning potential.
2. **Efficiency:** Optimize your time and resources to maximize productivity and profitability
3. **Entrepreneurship:** Cultivate an entrepreneurial mindset to identify and seize business opportunities
4. **Investment:** Understand and engage in wise investments to grow your wealth over time
5. **Networking:** Build and maintain professional relationships that can lead to new opportunities and collaborations
6. **Savings:** Implement effective saving strategies to ensure financial security and future investments
7. **Diversification:** Diversify your income streams to mitigate risks and ensure steady financial growth.

Expectation :

1. **Clarity:** Clearly define your expectations to avoid misunderstandings
2. **Realism:** Set realistic expectations based on circumstances and capabilities
3. **Communication:** Communicate your expectations clearly and openly with others
4. **Flexibility:** Be open to adjusting expectations as situations evolve
5. **Patience:** Understand that some expectations may take time to fulfil
6. **Empathy:** Consider others' perspectives and expectations in interactions
7. **Self-Awareness:** Reflect on your own expectations and how they influence your experiences.

|| ॐ ||

Shetall G Desai

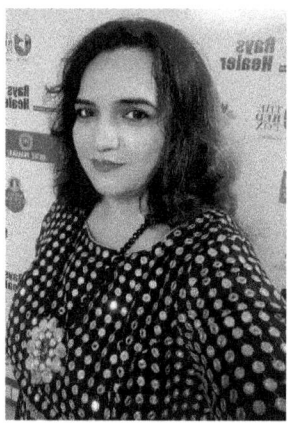

Author's Name	:	Shetall G Desai
Qualification	:	M.Com.
Current Profession	:	Practice in Occult Science
Age	:	42 years
E-mail ID	:	**sheetalgauravdesai81@gmail.com**
City/ Country	:	**Mumbai, India**

Shetall G Desai is a renowned Tarot Counselor, Numerologist, Candle Healer, Fengshui Consultant. She has clients all over the globe. She has won many awards for different modalities. She has learnt more than 20 modalities in occult science. She has not only changed her life but has changed lives of people around the globe. Serving society and helping them is the main goal of her life.

In the contemporary world, three pillars fundamentally shape our personal and professional trajectories; Learning, Earning, Expectation. Each of these are intervowen, influencing and reinforcing the others. Understanding the interplay between these three elements is crucial for navigating the complexities of modern life.

Learning :

Learning means acquiring skills and knowledge by study or by experience.

1. **Foundation:** Learning is the foundation of growth and corner stone for Human Development.
2. **Ongoing Process:** Learning is an ongoing process that begins from birth and continues throughout our lives. We learn from our mistakes too.

3. **Formal Education:** Schools, colleges and universities play a pivotal role in providing foundational knowledge and specialized training as they also foster critical thinking, creativity and social skills which are essential for personal and professional success.

4. **Lifelong Success:** The concept of lifelong learning emphasizes the need for continuos education and skill development, with rapid technological advancements and shifting job markets, individuals must continually update their knowledge to remain relevant and competitive.

5. **Informal Learning:** Learning also occurs outside the formal settings through experiences, observations and interactions is often self motivated and driven by curiosity and personal interests.

6. **Spiritual Learning:** When you elevate yourself through the power of your mind and start to live when you commit your life to cause higher than yourself.

7. **Drives Earning:** Learning drives Earning. Individuals who invest in their education and skills are often seen in having higher earning potential from various professions where advanced degrees and specialized training translate into better job oppurnities and higher salaries.

Earning :

1. **Learning:** Earning is instrinsically linked to learning

2. **Sustenance:** Earning is a direct consequence of applying this knowledge and skill in a market driven economy, providing the means for sustenance and advancement.

3. **Learning Drives Earning:** Individuals who invest in their education and skills often see higher earning potential in various professions where advanced degrees and specialized training translate into better job opportunities and higher salaries.

4. **Earning Meets Expectations:** Achieving financial stability and career success helps individuals meet both personal and societal expectations like respect, name, fame and goodwill.

5. **Rewards:** Financial rewards provide the means to pursue further learning and personal development, creating a positive feedback loop and non-financial rewards like blessings, warm and good wishes help us to heal our karmas and even give us a sense of satisfaction.

6. **Expectations Influence Learning:** Expectations, whether personal goals or societal standards, shape the learning paths individuals choose as high expectations can lead to greater efforts in education and skill acquisition, while unrealistic expectations can cause frustration and burnout.

7. **Blessings:** Blessings are the ways of our progress will definitely open up which helps us in achieving mental peace and harmony in our life.

Expectation :

1. **Perception:** Expectation is the lens through perception which individuals and societies gauge success, progress and satisfaction.

2. **Personal Expectations:** These are shaped by individual goals, values, and aspirations which drives self-improvement and the pursuit of excellence, influencing decisions about education, career paths, and lifestyle choices.

3. **Societal Expectations:** Society often sets benchmarks for success, such as educational attainment, career milestones, and material wealth as these expectations can inspire individuals to strive for higher achievements but can also create pressure to conform to societal norms.

4. **Managing Expectations:** Balancing personal and societal expectations is crucial for maintaining mental and emotional well-being as it involves setting realistic goals, recognizing one's limitations, and finding satisfaction in personal achievements rather than external validation.

5. **Humanitarian Expectations:** On human grounds it is always expected that we help each other in difficult times especially and it brings harmony around us for everyones well being .

6. **Disappointment:** Keeping too high expectations in life may create too many disappointments.

7. **Loyalty:** Exceeding expectation is where satisfaction ends and loyalty begins.

In conclusion, the interplay between learning, earning and expectation forms the bedrock of personal and professional development. Learning equips individuals with the necessary tools to succeed, earning provides the means to achieve stability and fulfillment, and expectations guide and motivate the pursuit of these goals. Understanding and balancing these elements are crucial for navigating life's challenges and achieving a harmonious and satisfying existence. As the world continues to evolve, the importance of adapting our learning, earning strategies and managing our expectations becomes ever more significant.

|| ॐ ||

Shikha Meher

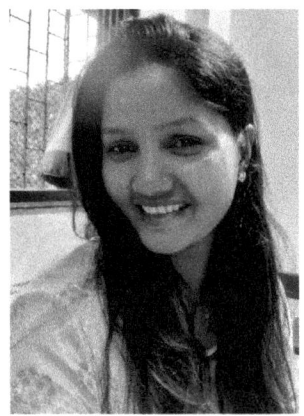

Author's Name	:	Shikha Meher
Qualification	:	H.S.C
Current Profession	:	Tarot Card Reader, Numerologist
Age	:	43 years
E-mail ID	:	**sheekhameher3@gmail.com**
City/ Country	:	**Mumbai, India**

Shikha Meher is a professional renowned for her expertise in tarot card reading, numerology, candle magic healing, crystal healing and remedies. With 6 years of dedicated experience in the occult field, she has positively transformed many people's lives through her accurate and insightful tarot readings. Her work in this field has guided individuals towards clarity, healing and personal growth.

In addition to her occult practice, Shikha has been a pet groomer for 15 years. Her extensive experience in pet grooming has allowed her to care for and enhance the well-being of countless pets. This dual expertise in both human and pet care highlights her commitment to improving lives, whether through spiritual guidance or practical grooming skills.

Shikha has the below LEEs of life :

Learning :

1. Learning is powerful weapon to solve all your problems
2. Learning is something we do get the knowledge of it

3. Learning can change goal of your life
4. Learning is self-improvement through education
5. Learning is method to update yourself
6. Learning is understanding financial concept
7. Learning may change your behavior towards your achievement

Earning :

1. Earning makes you powerful and decision maker
2. Earing is most important to live your life better
3. Earning person knows to survive in different situations
4. Earning is achieving victory
5. Earning is achieving financial stability and growth
6. Earning what we do for live our life
7. Earning can make you more powerful and strong

Expectation :

1. Expectation is better do with ourself
2. Expectiaton is what society want from us
3. Expectation is what we should not accept from others
4. Expectation is what we want others to do the way we want and it never happened
5. Expectation may set career goal and expecting
6. Expectation make you feel proud of yourself
7. Expectation may fulfill our own dream to reality

|| ॐ ||

Shipra Goswami

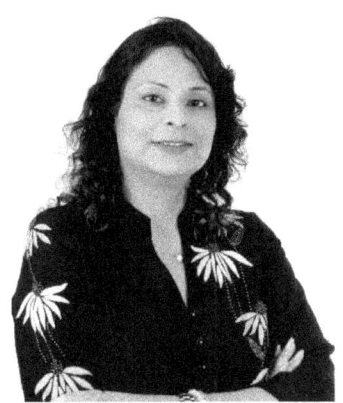

Author's Name	:	Shipra Goswami
Qualification	:	B.Com., M.B.A
Current Profession	:	Team Lead Business Development
Age	:	47 years
E-mail ID	:	**shipragoswami123@gmail.com**
City/ Country	:	**Gurgaon, India**

Shipra Goswami is a senior revenue development professional at Forrester, based in Gurgaon. She is responsible for managing India operations from last 11 years at Forrester. She has been awarded with many awards for her contribution in the field of excellence. She has done her graduation from Panjab University, Chandigarh and M.B.A from Delhi. Along with having a successful career she is a caring mother of twins and a dotted wife. She is a strong believer of God and Good Deeds.

In life, we learn valuable lessons that shape our experiences. Resilience teaches us to bounce back from setbacks, while empathy fosters deeper connections with others. Time management helps us prioritize effectively and financial literacy ensures stability. We also learn the importance of adaptability in an ever-changing world and the value of self-awareness in making informed decisions. As we navigate life, we earn significant qualities such as loyalty, respect and trust, which enrich our relationships. Our expectations include achieving personal fulfillment, attaining career success and maintaining a healthy work-life balance, all contributing to a meaningful and rewarding life.

Learning :

1. **Resilience:** Learning to bounce back from setbacks and challenges.
2. **Empathy:** Developing the ability to understand and share the feelings of others.
3. **Time Management:** Effectively managing time and prioritizing tasks is essential for achieving goals.
4. **Financial Literacy:** Learning about budgeting, saving, and investing.
5. **Adaptability:** Being able to adapt to change and embrace new experiences.
6. **Self-Awareness:** Understanding one's strengths, weaknesses, and values.
7. **Lifelong Learning:** Embracing the concept of continuous learning and growth.

Earning :

1. **Wisdom:** Gaining knowledge and insights from experiences.
2. **Love:** Cultivating deep emotional connections with others for support and joy.
3. **Gratitude:** life's blessings, fostering a positive outlook.
4. **Courage:** Gaining the strength to face fears and challenges.
5. **Self-Discipline:** Learning to control impulses and stay focused on long-term goals.
6. **Happiness:** Fulfillment and joy in everyday moments and achievements.
7. **Balance:** Achieving a healthy equilibrium between work, relationships, and personal time.

Expectation :

1. **Personal Fulfillment:** Joy and satisfaction in personal achievements and hobbies.
2. **Career Success:** Hard work will lead to professional advancement and recognition.
3. **Healthy Relationships:** Meaningful connections with family, friends, and partners.
4. **Financial Stability:** Level of financial security and independence.
5. **Good Health:** To maintain physical and mental well-being.
6. **Work-Life Balance:** To manage professional responsibilities while enjoying personal time.
7. **Continuous Growth:** To learn, evolve and adapt throughout life's challenges and experiences.

॥ ॐ ॥

Shweta Singh

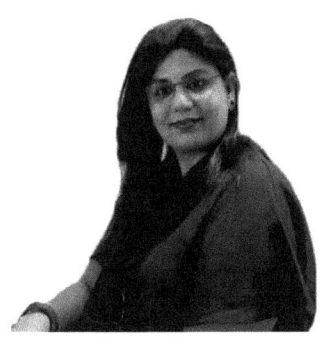

Author's Name	:	Shweta Singh
Qualification	:	B.B.A., B.Ed., M.B.A.
Current Profession	:	Consultant and Advisor
Age	:	45 Years
E-mail ID	:	**shwetasingh.vastugyan@gmail.com**
City/ Country	:	**Mumbai, India**

Shweta Singh is a renowned Shree Vastu Consultant and Certified Vedic Astrologer. She has done her Master Degree in Business Management and worked as Event Coordinator and a Teacher for many years in different schools in Gurgaon. She expanded her horizon of work and came into occult sciences to solve problems behind the scenes through Sanatan Principles of working such as Vastu Shastra, Vedic Astrology and Dousing.

She also is a creative spirit, who loves to paint, sketch and write. She coaches budding artists to fine tune their desire of expression through portraying on paper.

Life is a series of wisdom we amass over years which helps us live peacefully. Each experience, challenge or victory contributes to expand our understanding-guiding our decisions and actions.

With passing time, this collection of wisdom enables us to navigate through life's complexities with greater insight and purpose.

Each lesson, whether it's a triumph or a setback, contributes to our overall growth and perspective.

These hotchpotch incidents of life help us make sense of the external and internal world we live in and our place in the same. This journey of continuous learning and adaptation is a fundamental aspect of human development.

Learning :

1. **Health:** it's my best armour suit against adversity.
2. **Awareness:** what's going on around me is happening to me.
3. **Resourceful:** I should be on the list of others.
4. **Friends:** they have my back when I'm not ready.
5. **Money:** very important and it's easy to make enough of it by being skilled.
6. **Spiritual connect:** important to stay on the right course.
7. **Planet Earth:** plant more trees , it's our only place to be.

Earning :

1. **Mentors:** provide a strong grip on the roller coaster of life.
2. **Family:** keeps me going, my gas station to refuel.
3. **Vedic wisdom;** keeps me checked and on path towards my goal.
4. **Spirituality:** nurtures my soul and keeps my energy flowing.
5. **Knowing Self;** has helped me curate a path to walk on and live a purposeful life.
6. **Knowing** what I don't want shapes my goals and keeps me focused and speeds up achievements.
7. **Blessings;** keep me up float in tough times.

Expectation :

1. Wish I had a coach to look after my health and nourishment.
2. Wish I had more strengthen bonds with the universe for better intuition.
3. Wish I had invested in yoga clubs for deeper connect with self and society.
4. Wish I had met more mentors for richer insights.
5. Wish I had accepted what I could not change and used my precious time efficiently.
6. Wish I had met more people and talked to them about their lives.
7. Wish I had known this early that making money was the easiest thing and all I ever needed was a wish to make lots of it.

|| ॐ ||

Sri Rajeshwari Devi

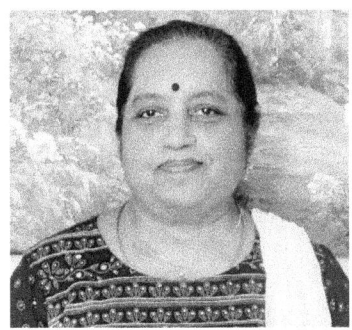

Author's Name	:	Sri Rajeshwari Devi
Qualification	:	M.A.(English), M.A. (Counseling Psychology)
Current Profession	:	Counseling Psychologist
Age	:	63 Years
E-mail ID	:	**authorsri60@gmail.com**
City/ Country	:	**Bangalore, India**

Sri Rajeshwari Devi is a Counseling Psychologist, Life skill Coach, Graphoanalytical Therapist and an Author. She has done her Master Degrees in English and Counseling Psychology, Diploma in Community Mental Health, Diploma in N.L.P and Certificate in Career Counseling. She has more than 16 years of experience as a Counseling Psychologist.

She is a Certified Career Counselor and Tarot Card Reader. She spends more of her leisure time reading, writing, traveling and giving emotional support to Cancer Patients and their relatives. She has published some of the articles in international science journals.

"Wisdom is not a product of schooling but of lifelong attempt to acquire it"

- Albert Einstein

Through this topic let us know about seven types of **Learning**, seven types of **Earning** and seven types of **Expectations** through which one can learn basic life skills.

Learning: Learning is a lifelong process by which individuals continuously gain new skills and knowledge. It is good for healthy body and mind, protecting us from Alzheimer or Dementia. It gives the people the skills to adopt, empowers to stay competitive in the job market and technological changes in their everyday life. According to UNESCO, the four pillars of Learning are 1) Learning to know (mind, body, emotions, intentions, expectation), 2) Learning to do, 3) Learning to be, and 4) Learning to live together.

Earning: Though earning money is the basic necessity of life, there are so many other things which has to be earned. Even though money helps us to achieve our goals, it cannot buy us love, good health or happiness.

Expectation: Expectations are essential since it gives a sense of achievement and a purpose of life. I believe one of the keys to happiness lies within the management of our expectations of people and circumstance. Unrealistic expectations like finding perfect career or perfect spouse etc. can lead to disappointment.

Learning :

1. Learning Mindfulness and living in the present helps to reduce stress.
2. Learning to set healthy Boundaries helps to find inner peace.
3. Learning from our own mistakes helps us to achieve biggest goals.
4. Learning to be adaptable is one of the best ways to win in life.
5. Learning to living our life to the fullest is the important life lesson.
6. Learning to forgive helps to improve our physical and mental health.
7. Learning to accept our flaws allow us to be happy than to be stressed.

Earning :

1. Earning good relationship with family and friends is one of the assets.
2. Earning good friends enrich your life and improve your health.
3. Earning respect develops strong relationship & opens door to new opportunities.
4. Earning trust needs lot of time and it demonstrates you are trustworthy.
5. Earning significance is acquired by doing something useful.
6. By Earning wisdom, we get profound understanding of life & people.
7. Earning efficiency with discipline, persistence & practice improves health.

Expectation :

1. Expecting imperfection in relationships is the key to make perfect relationship
2. Expecting imperfection in situation is an act of self-love and acceptance.
3. Expect that we should never have arguments, since arguing is toxic.
4. Expecting that you can change someone is highly impossible.
5. Expecting the family members to spend some time together helps to strengthen the bonds between family members.
6. It is better to stop expecting everyone should agree with us
7. Expecting the partner not to disrespect may be pointless.

|| ॐ ||

Sudha Krishnan

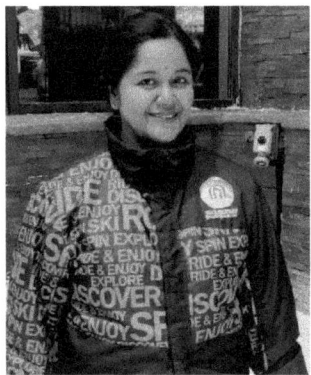

Author's Name	:	Sudha Krishnan
Qualification	:	B.Com.
Current Profession	:	Healer and Handwriting Analyst
Age	:	56 years
E-mail ID	:	**krishnansudha9@gmail.com**
City/ Country	:	**Hyderabad, India**

Sudha Krishnan, originally from Mumbai and now residing in Hyderabad, has 24 years of experience in a Nationalized Bank. She is a Healer and a trained Handwriting Analyst, utilizing her unique skills in handwriting therapy and various healing modalities to help others achieve personal growth and well-being. Sudha is also deeply committed to animal welfare, a passion that began in Tamil Nadu, where she started caring for stray dogs. Now, she dedicates time to feeding and providing medical care for strays in her community.

Sudha balances her professional life with being a mother to two grown-up children and a devoted caregiver to her beloved dog, Cookie.

This article is a comprehensive guide to living a meaningful and balanced life, framed around the principles of Learning, Earning and Expectation. It blends spiritual wisdom with practical advice, urging readers to make God their guiding force, respect their parents, and nurture their relationships with love and compassion. It underscores the importance of integrity, self-care, and high-frequency living. This article also explores how to earn love, blessings, and greatness through virtuous actions, while maintaining clarity through prayer and meditation. It concludes with insights on embracing success, freedom, forgiveness, and personal growth, fostering a life of equality and effective communication.

Learning :

1) **Spiritual:** Make God your Guru and your nearest and dearest.
2) **Parents:** Respect your parents and always be there for them.
3) **Connection:** Communicate and be connected to your family members, siblings, close friends and relatives.
4) **Serve:** Help and ask help.
5) **Values:** Be a leader with integrity, commitment and compassion.
6) **Health:** Respect and take care of your body and mind.
7) **Smile:** Always vibrate at a high frequency

Earning :

1) **Love:** Earn lots of love
2) **Blessings:** Earn blessings through good deeds
3) **Greatness:** Earn greatness through learnings and experiences.
4) **Health:** Earn good health by eating right and exercise.
5) **Clarity:** Earn a clear mind through prayer and meditation.
6) **Respect:** Earn respect by giving respect and doing your duty.
7) **Wealth:** Earn wealth by hard work, dedication and wisdom.

Expectation :

1) **Success:** To do well in life.
2) **Freedom:** To live and let live.
3) **Love:** Forgive and forget.
4) **Nothingness:** Surrender to the divine.
5) **Equality:** To treat all as one.
6) **Connect:** To communicate right.
7) **Growth:** To grow and accept change

॥ ॐ ॥

Suvigya Seraphim Raj

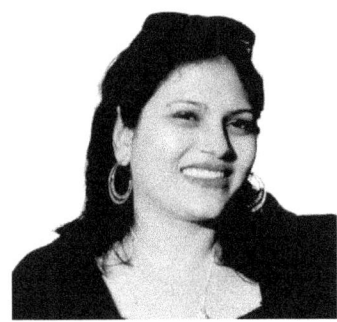

Author's Name	:	Suvigya Seraphim Raj
Qualification	:	MBA (Human Resources and Marketing)
Current Profession	:	Sr. HR Consultant/ Talent Advisor
Age	:	42 years
E-mail ID	:	**contactsr21@gmail.com**
City/ Country	:	**Toronto, Cañada**

Suvigya Seraphim Raj is a Sr. HR Consultant working with a top US global recruitment process outsourcing company. She holds a Master's Degrees in Business Administration from Mount Carmel Institute of Management, Bangalore, India. She is deeply committed to helping clients discover top IT/ Engineering professionals for consulting engagements. Her unwavering dedication revolves around the genuine well-being and success of both consultants and clients alike.

Suvigya has the below LEEs of life :

Learning :

1. **Optimism -** Nurturing and strengthening optimism is a core theme in my life and work.
2. **Pace Yourself-Slow down**—don't rush into things. Let your life unfold. Wait a bit to see where it takes you and take time to weigh your options.
3. **You can't please everyone -** You don't need everyone to agree with you or even be like you. It's human nature to want to belong, to be liked, respected, and valued, but not at the expense of your integrity and happiness.
4. **Health -** Health is an invaluable treasure—always appreciate, nurture, and protect it.

5. **Life Expectations** - No matter how carefully you plan and how hard you work, sometimes things just don't work out the way you want them to... and that's okay.

6. **Love** - Love is not just a feeling; it's a choice that you make every day. We have to choose to let annoyances pass, to forgive, to be kind, to respect, to support, to be faithful.

7. **Patience** - In life, you'll have to wait for a lot of things without feeling negative.

Earning :

1. **Family** - I have a beautiful family that I cherish every day.

2. **Spirituality** - Healthy *spirituality* gives a sense of peace, wholeness and balance among the physical, emotional, social and **spiritual** aspects of our lives.

3. **Relationship** - Nurture your family relationships, these will be the people that will be there for you.

4. **Friends** - I have friends I can trust with my life, and they are someone who have seen the best and worst of me and will be there whenever I need to talk to.

5. **Education** - I am grateful to my parents for providing me the best education. For making me what I am today, I can never thank them enough.

6. **Home** - I have a home which is a secure shelter for me and my loved ones.

7. **Job** - I express gratitude to God, family, and friends for my job.

Expectation :

1. **Success** - I will try to bring what little good I can, If I succeed, great! Happy by default. If I fail, its no one else to blame, I got the chance.

2. **Love** - We know that love is an important element for achieving happiness.

3. **Family Happiness** - My family is my life and everything else comes second. I want my family to be happy and healthy.

4. **Respect** - The thing which I really expect from life is respect. And I have learnt from my past and mistakes that life won't give me respect just like that. You have to give respect to earn it.

5. **Fruitful Journey** - I expect life to be a fruitful journey. A lot of the older generations have said that each of us has a purpose here on Earth, and the reason for our existence is to complete that purpose.

6. **Changes** - I expect life will be unpredictable. Like many others, I have learned that things don't always go as you planned and have started accepting changes.

7. **Professional** - Obtaining a job that makes me happy and financial stable, as well as helping the less fortunate.

|| ॐ ||

Suyog Patil

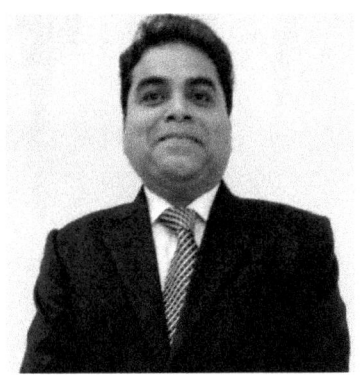

Author's Name	:	Suyog Patil
Qualification	:	Bachelor Degree in Science, M.B.A.
Current Profession	:	Entrepreneur and Consultant
Age	:	48 years
E-mail ID	:	suyog_p2@rediffmail.com
City/ Country	:	**Mumbai, India**

Suyog Patil is an Entrepreneur, Consultant, Graphologist, Face Reader, Angel Therapist, Akashic Reader and a Writer. He has done his Graduation in Science and Masters in Business Management. He has worked for 22 years in Seven Companies including Corporates like Pidilite and MNC's. He is a Partner with Ariel Engineering and Technologies and Proprietor of Standard Vacuum Industries.

Suyog's Father and Grandfather had their own Photo Studios, but His Passion since Childhood was to join The Indian Airforce, but couldn't make it and opted for his second carrier choice of completing Masters in Business Management. Had decided to get into full time Business only after gaining sufficient Rich Work Experience and designated his carrier in that Path.

He is a Happy, Joyful Person who believes in Spirituality and Practices the same.

Learning Earning and Expectations are one of the main Aspects of Life for which we Live our Life and walk on the Progress Path of Life. Learning teaches us how to take our Journey of Life by Learning New Things each and every Day. Who is a Student? Answer is Every Human Being is a Student as we learn something New Each and Every Day. Learning leads us to Earnings and Expectations in our Life Journey. Proper Learning leads to proper Earning and our Learning and Earnings leads to proper Investments and our Earnings and Investments Fulfils are Expectations in

Life. When we fulfil our Expectations in Life we feel Happy, Joys, Satisfied and Successful in Life. To conclude Learning, Earning and Expectations are related with each other.

Learning :

1) **Endless:** There is no end to your learning, new learning and relearning is a process of your entire life.

2) **Every Day:** In Your Life Journey you learn something new every day.

3) **Guidance:** Learning should be taken as Guidance for Life.

4) **Motivational:** Every Day Learning should be a motivation for Life Path.

5) **Correction:** Learning should be a corrective measure for our past mistakes.

6) **Mistake:** Whenever You make mistake in life take it as Learning Experience so that you do not repeat the same again.

7) **Abundance:** Learning should be used in a proper way to bring Abundance of Knowledge in Life.

Earning :

1) **Earning:** Earning should me minimum Four Times than your Spending.

2) **Spending:** Only Small Amount of Earning should be spent.

3) **Investments:** Investments of Majority Earnings should be done in such a way that in Long Term the Returns are Multifold.

4) **Abundance:** Earnings should bring in Abundance flow of Income in Life.

5) **Multisource:** Earnings should be from Multiple sources so that the Expansion in Investments become Faster.

6) **Multifold:** Earnings should be Multifold to Increase the Wealth.

7) **Gratitude:** Earning should be welcomed in Life with Gratitude.

Expectation :

1) **Successful:** To be successful Spiritually and Mentally.

2) **Abundance:** Abundance Money wise, Health wise

3) **Family:** Family should be Loving, Caring and Understanding each other Family Members and their views.

4) **Spouse:** Spouse should be such a person who is matured enough to handle each and every situation in Married Life.

5) **Maturity:** One should handle situations and challenges that arouse in Life in a Matured way day by day.

6) **Peacful:** Entire Life Journey should be a peaceful Journey. This is possible if one gives time for a low phase to pass through Life Cycle.

7) **Expectations:** Life should be full of Abundance, Love, Joy and Happiness.

॥ ॐ ॥

Tanvee Kakati

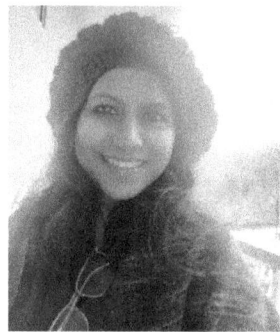

Author's Name	:	Tanvee Kakati
Qualification	:	M.A. (Sociology) Visharad in Vocals, NLP, Ho'oponopono healing, LOA and Energy Coaching, CBT, Happiness coach, Reiki, Mental Health counseling, Meditation Teacher
Current Profession	:	Consultant, Energy coach and Singer
Age	:	35 years
E-mail ID	:	**harmonywithtanvee@gmail.com**
City/ Country	:	**Guwahati, India**

Tanvee Kakati, originally from Guwahati, Assam, is rooted in a culturally rich family of artists. She graduated in sociology from the prestigious Hindu College and the Delhi School of Economics, University of Delhi. She has also cleared the UGC- NET and has been invited as guest speaker in colleges. With nearly a decade of experience, Tanvee has worked as a researcher, consultant and program manager on social impact projects for esteemed non-profit organisations and research institutions like MIT (USA) and the University of Surrey. She has led initiatives funded by organizations such as UNDP, the US Embassy, DFID. etc in some renowned organisations. Additionally, Tanvee is a passionate trained singer, with her regional songs featured on AIR Guwahati.

Besides this, her love for human development has guided her to specialize in positive psychology and energy healing, utilizing techniques like CBT, reiki and NLP. She has studied under notable teachers, including Eckhart Tolle and Deepak Chopra. Currently, she is pursuing mind and energy coaching, believing that life is an art. An avid traveller, Tanvee views the world as her home and seeks spiritual growth through her journeys.

Embracing LEE has profoundly shaped my journey. It reminds me to savor lessons learned, celebrate both tangible and intangible rewards, and nurture my aspirations. Together, these elements foster resilience, purpose, and a deeper sense of connection, enabling us to navigate challenges and celebrate successes while living a meaningful and conscious life. Knowing the seven LEE of life has made me more grounded. By integrating these principles, I find deeper presence, fulfillment, balance, and connection, enriching my life's path.

'**LEE**' Learning, Earning and Expectations; represents a holistic framework for living a fulfilled and evolving life.

Learning encompasses continuous growth through education and experiences, shaping our understanding and skills.

Earning refers to both financial stability and the intangible rewards of personal efforts, fostering a sense of accomplishment.

Expectations set the standards for what we seek in life, guiding our goals and aspirations.

To me, '**LEE**' serves as a guiding light for my life. It reflects my commitment to continuous self-discovery, the pursuit of meaningful accomplishments, and the cultivation of relationships that inspire growth and joy in every moment.

Learning :

1. **Self-Awareness**: Understanding your thoughts, emotions, and motivations helps you navigate life more effectively.
2. **Embrace Change**: Life is full of transitions, and adapting to change fosters resilience and growth.
3. **The Importance of Relationships**: Nurturing meaningful connections enhances happiness and support during tough times.
4. **Practice Gratitude**: Focusing on what you appreciate shifts your mindset and increases overall well-being.
5. **Learn from Failure**: Mistakes and setbacks are opportunities for growth and learning; they pave the way for success.
6. **Mindfulness**: Being present helps you enjoy the moment and reduces anxiety about the future.
7. **Pursue Passion**: Engaging in what you love brings fulfillment and purpose, making life more rewarding.

Earning :

1. **Wisdom**: Gained through life experiences, reflection, and learning, wisdom enriches decision-making and perspective.
2. **Emotional Resilience**: The ability to navigate challenges and recover from setbacks enhances personal strength and mental well-being.

3. **Inner Peace**: Cultivating a sense of calm and contentment fosters stability and fulfillment, regardless of external circumstances.

4. **Authentic Relationships**: Building genuine connections with others contributes to emotional support, belonging, and a sense of community.

5. **Self-Awareness**: Understanding one's thoughts, feelings, and motivations deepens personal insight and enhances interpersonal interactions.

6. **Spiritual Growth**: Engaging in practices that nurture the spirit, such as meditation or mindfulness, leads to a greater sense of purpose and connectedness.

7. **Creativity**: Developing and expressing creativity through art, writing, or other forms fosters self-expression and personal fulfillment.

Expectation :

1. **Fulfillment**: A desire to find meaning and purpose in personal and professional endeavors.

2. **Happiness**: An expectation to experience joy, contentment, and positive emotions throughout life.

3. **Growth**: The belief that life should provide opportunities for personal and professional development.

4. **Connection**: An expectation for meaningful relationships with family, friends, and community.

5. **Adventure**: A desire for new experiences, travel, and exploration that enrich life.

6. **Balance**: The expectation to maintain a healthy balance between work, leisure, passion and personal time.

7. **Harmony**: An expectation to cultivate balance and peace within oneself and in relationships, fostering a sense of unity with the world.

|| ॐ ||

Tejjal Bhanshalii

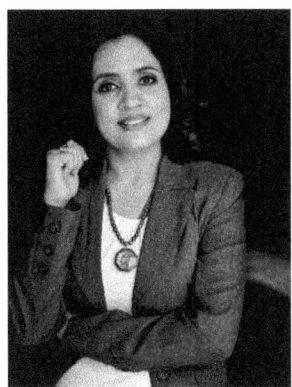

Author's Name	:	Tejjal Bhanshalii
Qualification	:	Nutritionist 20 Yrs Practice
Current Profession	:	Psychic and Holistic Healer
Age	:	42 Years
E-mail ID	:	**tejuritu5454@gmail.com**
City/ Country	:	**New Delhi, India**

Tejjal Bhanshalii is a passionate advocate of holistic healing through a variety of modalities. Her practice encompasses Access Bars, intuitive healing and distance healing, each designed to dissolve energy blockages and foster mental clarity. She specializes in chakra balancing and aura cleansing, essential for maintaining energetic harmony and vitality. Through talk therapy and word energy techniques, She facilitates emotional release and mental well-being, guiding individuals towards inner peace and resilience.

Tejjal's mission is to empower individuals on their healing journeys, helping them discover the interconnectedness of mind, body, and spirit. With compassion and expertise, She strives to create a supportive environment, where healing and self-discovery flourish.

In a world filled with constant noise and distraction, it's easy to get caught up in the mundane and overlook the profound. Life's journey is often viewed through a narrow lens, shaped by societal expectations and personal fears. But what if we dared to explore beyond the surface? What if we sought out the hidden dimensions of existence that are waiting to be discovered? This article is an invitation to step off the beaten path and delve into the uncharted territories of life—where true transformation and enlightenment await.

The journey through life is much more than a series of predictable events. It's a dynamic process of unfolding, where every experience—pleasant or painful—carries the potential for transformation. To truly live, we must be willing to explore the unknown, to question the status quo, and to find meaning in the unexpected. This understanding of life is not just an intellectual exercise; it's a way of being that resonates deeply with the soul

Learning :

1. **Beyond Academia**: True learning happens in life's quiet moments, beyond the confines of formal education.
2. **Embrace Failure**: Failure is not a setback but a stepping stone to greater wisdom.
3. **Life as a Teacher**: Every experience, whether good or bad, teaches us something valuable about ourselves and the world.
4. **Inner Silence**: Real insights come in moments of stillness, where the mind is free to explore the unknown.
5. **Continuous Growth**: Learning is a lifelong journey; we must remain open to new ideas and perspectives.
6. **Courage to Question**: Challenge the norms and ask difficult questions to uncover deeper truths.
7. **Embody Knowledge**: It's not just about acquiring knowledge but integrating it into our lives and actions.

Earning :

1. **Beyond Money**: Earning isn't just about financial gain; it's about accumulating experiences and insights.
2. **Wealth of Relationships**: The true measure of wealth lies in the depth and quality of our relationships.
3. **Internal Richness**: Cultivate inner peace and contentment as the ultimate form of earning.
4. **Value of Time**: Invest your time wisely; it's a currency that cannot be replenished.
5. **Soul Enrichment**: Seek out experiences that nourish the soul, not just the wallet.
6. **Purpose Over Profit**: Align your earnings with your life's purpose for deeper fulfillment.
7. **Legacy of Wisdom**: What we earn in life is not just material but the wisdom we leave behind for others.

Expectation :

1. **Fluidity of Life**: Life rarely follows a strict plan; embrace its unpredictable nature.
2. **Release Control**: Let go of rigid expectations; they often lead to disappointment.
3. **Trust the Process**: Believe that every detour is guiding you to where you're meant to be.
4. **Unexpected Gifts**: Often, the most meaningful experiences come from what we least expect.

5. **Open to Change**: Be flexible and adapt to new circumstances as they arise.

6. **Serendipity**: Allow room for spontaneity and unexpected opportunities.

7. **Faith in the Journey**: Have faith that the path you're on is the right one, even if it diverges from your original plan.

Life is an uncharted path, full of hidden dimensions that are waiting to be explored. It's a journey that requires us to go beyond the ordinary and to seek out the extraordinary in every moment. By embracing the unknown, by learning, earning, and expecting in ways that go beyond the conventional, we open ourselves to a life of profound depth and meaning. The true essence of life lies not in what we achieve, but in how we evolve through each experience, how we transform through each challenge, and how we find enlightenment in the most unexpected places

॥ ॐ ॥

Trina Kanungo

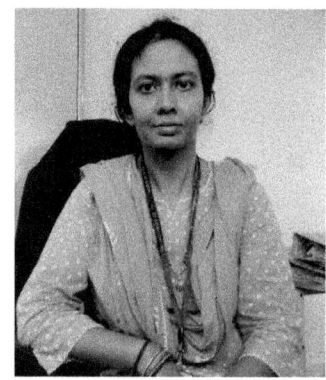

Author's Name	:	Trina Kanungo
Qualification	:	M.Sc. (Maths & Computing-IIT Dhanbad)
Current Profession	:	Scale 2 Officer, ECGC Ltd, under Ministry of Commerce
Age	:	31 years
E-mail ID	:	...
City/ Country	:	**Mumbai, India**

Trina Kanungo, hailing from Hind Motor, West Bengal, a Postgraduate in Mathematics and Computing from IIT Dhanbad, currently serves as an Assistant Manager (Scale 2 Officer) at ECGC Ltd. in Mumbai, under the Ministry of Commerce and Industry, Government of India. Beyond her professional role, Trina's passions lie in Indian Fine Arts, Yoga and Literature.

Trina's literary contributions shine brightly, being a co-author of numerous anthologies in English and Bengali literature. Her literary prowess has been recognized through multiple awards and accolades. She has been awarded Honorary Doctorate on "Peace and Meditation" by the Grace Ladies Global Academy, USA, in the year 2022 for her tireless contribution to the society towards fitness goals through yoga and meditation.

In my life, **Learning** fuels personal and professional growth, offering knowledge and skills that open doors to new opportunities and understanding. **Earning** come in many forms, from financial stability to the richness of meaningful relationships and health. **Expectation** shapes our goals and aspirations, driving us to seek success, fulfillment, and balance. Balancing learning, earnings, and expectations involves setting realistic goals, adapting to change, and finding satisfaction in progress and achievements. By integrating these elements thoughtfully, we navigate life's complexities and create a fulfilling and purposeful existence .

Learning :

1) **Resilience**: Life always presents challenges and setbacks,learning to bounce back from adversity is what important for us.

2) **Gratitude**: Cultivating gratitude allows us to appreciate the good aspects in our lives, even amidst challenges.

3) **Empathy**: Understanding and empathizing with others' perspectives and emotions promotes kindness.

4) **Continuous Learning**: Embracing a mindset of lifelong learning keeps our minds active and adaptable to any adverse situation

5) **Self-compassion**: Being kind to ourselves in moments of failure or difficulty is crucial for maintaining mental and emotional health quotient.

6) **Adaptability**: Flexibility allows us to thrive in uncertain times and make the most of unforeseen opportunities.

7) **Purpose**: Having a sense of purpose gives our lives meaning and direction

Earning :

1) **Knowledge and Wisdom**: This includes formal education, life experiences, and personal decisions.

2) **Relationships and Communication skills**: Building strong, supportive relationships with family, friends, colleagues, and mentors provides and creates a sense of belonging and community.

3) **Health and Well-being**: Maintaining physical, mental, and emotional health is very significant.

4) **Financial Stability**: Achieving financial stability and security can offer peace of mind, the ability to pursue personal goals, and the freedom to make choices aligned with one's values and desires.

5) **Personal Growth and Fulfillment**: Pursuing passions, hobbies, and personal development contributes to a sense of achievement and satisfaction.

6) **Career Achievement**: Finding a career that aligns with one's skills and interests, can provide a sense of purpose and accomplishment.

7) **Legacy and Impact**: Contributing positively to the world and creating something lasting, allows individuals to leave a meaningful impact and be remembered for their contributions.

Expectation :

1) **Personal Success** :This could involve reaching specific milestones, gaining recognition, or realizing long-held dreams.

2) **Health and Wellness**: Individuals should expect to maintain good health and well-being throughout their lives.

3) **Work-Life Balance**: This involves having time for family, leisure activities, and self-care, while also fulfilling professional obligations.

4) **Financial Security:** This involves earning a reliable income, saving for the future, and managing finances responsibly.

5) **Fulfillment in Relationships**: This involves mutual respect, understanding, and shared values.

6) **Happiness:** This can be influenced by various factors, including personal achievements, relationships, and overall life satisfaction.

7) **Personal Growth and Learning**: Many expect to continue growing and learning throughout their lives. This can involve acquiring new skills, exploring new interests, and evolving as an individual.

॥ ॐ ॥

Uman Hooda

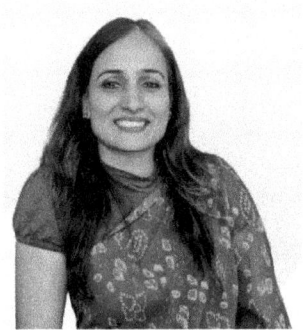

Author's Name	:	Uman Hooda
Qualification	:	M.C.A.
Current Profession	:	Microsoft Corporate Trainer and Consultant, Motivational speaker
Age	:	43 years
E-mail ID	:	**uman.kumari@gmail.com**
City/ Country	:	**Gurugram, India**

Uman Hooda is a Microsoft Certified Trainer (MCT) & Microsoft Certified Data Analyst. She has experience of working with Power BI, Power Platform, MS Dynamics and Azure. She has trained professionals and done consultancy projects around the globe.

She has previously worked as a Software Quality Analyst in multinational companies. She is a very impressive motivational speaker as well. She has motivated lots of people by listing their problems, doubts and giving some guidance to change and become better at living a happy life with peace.

Life is a journey and everyone experiences it in their own unique way. Each person has a different perspective on living, with varied interests and ambitions. We all have our own lessons, experiences, and expectations. I believe in lifelong learning and strive to find something good in everyone I meet. It's important to share our experiences and support others in any way we can, making their lives happier and more meaningful. Our lives reflect our minds—our thoughts, decisions, and the kind of person we are, shaped by our feelings, emotions, and experiences.

My guiding principle is, *"Everything happens for a good reason in life."*

Learning :

1. **Ambitious**: Set realistic goals with determination and take the necessary steps to achieve them. Without goals, life can feel meaningless.

2. **Humble, Kind & Forgiveness:** Kindness keeps us grounded, and forgiveness strengthens us by freeing us from holding grudges.

3. **Gratitude**: Being thankful for what we have is essential. Gratitude brings peace and relaxation.

4. **Punctuality & Discipline**: A punctual and disciplined approach is key to achieving success in life.

5. **Education and Financial Independence:** Education paves the way for a happy life. Everyone should strive for good education and financial security.

6. **Don't set expectations from others**: we should focus on self-reliance and manage our own expectations. It will give us the ability to understand other's perspective too.

7. **Know your abilities and have self-confidence**: we should recognize our strengths and believe in yourself.

Earning :

1. **Trust**: I've built trust with family and friends through honesty and reliability.

2. **Respect**: I've earned respect by valuing others and acting with integrity.

3. **Friendship**: I cultivate friendships through mutual support and empathy.

4. **Good Relationships:** The people in our lives are important. Good relationships contribute to happiness, health, and well-being.

5. **Happy Family Life**: A happy family is a blessing. Strong family bonds are built through love and communication.

6. **Financial Security**: Financial stability is crucial. I've achieved this through smart planning and saving.

7. **Positive Attitude**: I strive to see the positive in everything. This attitude has brought me success and attracted more positivity into my life, thanks to my life experiences.

Expectation :

1. **Health**: Health is wealth, and this is my top priority. With good health, anything is possible.

2. **Contributing to Social Services**: I expect myself to contribute more to social services, as it brings me deep satisfaction.

3. **Becoming a Successful Motivational Speaker: I** aspire to be a renowned motivational speaker, helping and inspiring others to live happy lives.

4. **Raising a Happy and Successful Daughter:** I want to raise my daughter to be a good human being who is happy, successful, and knows how to live a fulfilling life.

5. **Traveling and Exploring the World:** I love traveling and experiencing new cultures. I want to explore beautiful places around the world.

6. **Living a Satisfied Life**: Contentment is central to my life. I aim to always be happy and satisfied with what I have.

7. **Staying Active and Learning New Skills**: Staying active and continuously learning new skills keeps us motivated and excited. Learning is a lifelong process that should always be nurtured.

॥ ॐ ॥

Vaishali S Iyer

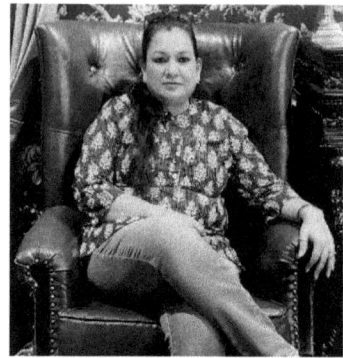

Author's Name	:	Vaishali S Iyer
Qualification	:	M.A. (English Literature)
Current Profession	:	Freelance Interlocutor for Cambridge Exams
Age	:	43 years
E-mail ID	:	**vaishali.s.iyer@gmail.com**
City/ Country	:	**Ahmedabad, India**

Vaishali S Iyer is a homemaker, a Freelancer and a Vastu practitioner. She has rich experience in Human Resources and content writing with more than 10+ years of experience in different domains. She works as a Freelancer for multiple organisations. Along with her Master's degree, she also holds various certifications from Cambridge Language Tests and has certificates from Vastu Shastra, Numerology and many more. Her love towards occult science has inclined her towards learning more about the subject and is still diving deep into other occult modalities.

The book here depicts seven aspects of life including our Learning, Earning and Expectation from life. We have seven chakras in the human body and each chakra has its importance and significance. The way we unfold each layer or chakra we tend to move forward in an upward direction. The same is true with life, once we start unfolding the secrets of our existence, we start moving in an upward direction towards liberation. Here, I have expressed my thoughts in a simple manner for the reader to understand.

Learning :

1. **Faith:** Have faith in yourself and the almighty.
2. **Discipline:** Significant for a successful life.

3. **Attitude:** A positive attitude towards everything always helps in difficult situations.
4. **Forgiveness:** Forgive people more often for your inner peace.
5. **Strength:** Be mentally and emotionally strong to face any turbulence in life.
6. **Patience:** Have patience at any given point of time, this will help you to tackle situations and people in a better manner.
7. **Advise:** Do not advise if it is not required. Advise only when you are asked to do so.

Earning :

1. **Skills:** Upgrade with more skills to evolve constantly.
2. **Values:** The most important thing for a human being is their values. Don't lose it.
3. **Education:** No one can steal this from you.
4. **Creativity:** The ability to do things creatively is an art.
5. **Dignity:** Always live with dignity and pass on the same to the next generation.
6. **Blessings:** Earn it through your good deeds and karma.
7. **Motherhood:** Bringing two beautiful souls into this world and nurturing them with good values and compassion for other living beings is the greatest earning for me till now.

Expectation :

1. **Success:** I want success in all aspects of my life.
2. **Health:** I want me and my family to be healthy always.
3. **Family:** I am grateful for all relationships in my life and always want them to be happy and prosperous.
4. **Travel:** I want to travel to different countries with my family. Travelling is like a therapy.
5. **Abundance:** I want abundance in my life, not just material but spiritual.
6. **Recognition:** I want to be recognised for the work I do.
7. **Nature:** Me and my family are nature lovers. We cherish nature and would love to do something on a large scale for Mother Nature as a sign of Gratitude! I hope these wishes get fulfilled soon.

|| ॐ ||

Veena Chugh

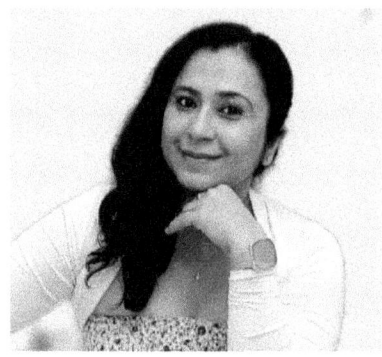

Author's Name	:	Veena Chugh
Qualification	:	B.Com., M.B.A.
Current Profession	:	Author, Coach, Public Speaker & Entrepreneur
Age	:	46 years
E-mail ID	:	**chugh.veena@gmail.com**
City/ Country	:	**United States of America**

Veena Chugh is the author of "A Pink Rose and Other Short Stories", a collection that reflects her spiritual journey and personal insights. With two decades of professional experience, Veena has held leadership roles, including serving as the Head of HR in her last two positions. She is also a certified yoga instructor, coach, and public speaker who advocates for mental health and personal development through holistic practices. Veena is the founder of "Arthaa Advisors" a consulting firm that supports individuals and families with wealth planning and legacy management. She has also served as visiting faculty at leading colleges in Mumbai.

Originally from Mumbai, Veena now lives in Conshohocken, Pennsylvania, with her husband and son. In her free time, she enjoys writing and exploring new recipes, drawing inspiration from both her professional and personal life.

The *'Seven LEE of Life'* – Learning, Earning and Expectation – are principles I hold dear, guiding me as both a writer and a person. Learning has been a constant companion, teaching me that being true to myself is where peace lies. Earning, for me, is about more than financial success; it's the memories I create, the smiles I inspire, and the peace I find within. It's knowing that each day brings the chance to earn something more valuable than money—fulfillment, love, and purpose. Expectations, too, have shaped my path. I've learned to set high standards for myself, but also to let go of perfectionism and embrace life's unpredictability. In the end, these seven principles remind me that life is a beautiful journey of growth, and I'm here to embrace every twist and turn with grace and gratitude.

Learning :

1. Be yourself— it lightens the weight you carry.
2. Love yourself unconditionally— it's the foundation for all growth.
3. Forgive easily— but never forget the wisdom gained.
4. Success has no shortcuts— enjoy every step of the journey.
5. Dream big— dreams have the power to take you to unimaginable places.
6. Kindness never goes out of fashion— be kind always.
7. Integrity grounds you— honor it every time, all the time.

Earning :

1. Time is your most precious asset— use it wisely.
2. Memories with loved ones are true wealth— cherish them.
3. A smile you create is a daily earning— value it.
4. Spend with good intentions— it nurtures an abundant mindset.
5. Peace of mind and love in your heart— these are your true riches.
6. Your mind is a powerful tool— use it to your advantage.
7. Strive daily to become your best self— because at the end, it's you with you

Expectation :

1. Gratitude protects against complacency— embrace it.
2. Expect the most from yourself— and work to meet it.
3. Evaluate others' expectations— honor what aligns with you, and address what doesn't.
4. Communication is key— to managing expectations effectively.
5. Always have a Plan B— for life's unforeseen challenges.
6. Unlearn perfectionism— it's a burden, not a goal.
7. Life's purpose is growth— and it may not follow your plans.

|| ॐ ||

Veenu Mehendiratta

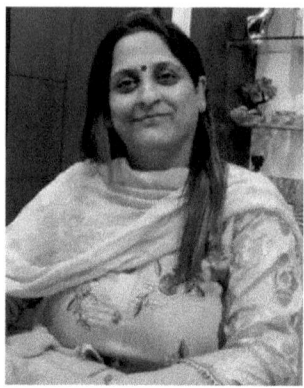

Author's Name	:	Veenu Mehendiratta
Qualification	:	Graduate
Current Profession	:	Occultist (veenumero)
Age	:	45 years
E-mail ID	:	**veenumero@gmail.com**
City/ Country	:	**Gwalior, India**

Mrs. Veenu Mehendiratta is an Occultist by passion and profession. She is a Numerologist, Tarot Card Reader, Dowsing Expert, Fortune Teller by Dice, Switch Words and Healing Codes Master. Have an expertise over Mind Money Mastery, a certified Life Coach and a Reiki Grand Master. From being a teacher turned into an industrialist, then from there, she moved towards being a home maker and devoted her time in growing kids and now at this phase, she has started her journey of being an Occultist. She always believes that whenever a person approaches any Occult practitioner, he or she is looking for the guidance and consider us the mediator that whatever we are going to tell him is the message from universe for him/ her, So, She always believes in showing the right and positive path to the native.

Mrs. Veenu feels blessed as universe has chosen her for the same.

The **'Seven LEE's of Life'** reflect the learning, earning and expectation that shape our journey. When I think back on my life, it's like watching a movie of my memories, from childhood to the present. I recall the lessons I've learned along the way, the things I've held onto, and what I hope the future will bring.

Learning goes beyond formal education. They come from the stories of our lives, shaped by the people we meet and the experiences we go through—both good and bad. These lessons build our belief systems, emotional and mental strength, decision-making abilities, social standing, relationships, and even financial gains. What we earn from these experiences influences our expectations for the future, determining whether we can meet them.

When I talk about expectations, it's like looking at the path ahead. I hope for love from those around me, dream of material success, and seek happiness in all aspects of life. But it's crucial to approach these expectations with the understanding that life can be unpredictable. Balancing what I've learned, earned, and expect from life is key to navigating whatever comes next.

Learning :

1. **Wisdom-** Accumulate knowledge from everything that's happening in your life.
2. **Change-** Life constantly changes from good times to bad and back again.
3. **Gratitude-** Expressing gratitude for everything can increase our happiness.
4. **Self-care-** It's important to prioritize self-care and honor the life you've been given.
5. **Kindness-** Kindness is the key to enriching your life and bring happiness.
6. **Honesty-** Be honest to yourself and lead a fulfilling life.
7. **Adaptability-** I have learned to adapt to every circumstance and change with a positive attitude.

Earning :

1. **Happiness -** I have cherished many happy and precious moments throughout every phase of my life.
2. **Success -** I have witnessed success in many personal and professional goals.
3. **Health -** The biggest earning of my life is my emotional health.
4. **Strength -** life's challenges and learnings have made me strong.
5. **Relationship -** I have formed relationships based on personal choice rather than just family ties.
6. **Trust -** I have been lucky enough to earn the trust of others.
7. **Abundance -** I have achieved abundance in every aspect of my life.

Expectation :

1. **Love -** I hope people will continue to love me for who I am.
2. **Growth -** I look forward to growing both personally and as a good human being.
3. **Respect -** I expect to be treated with respect.
4. **Stability -** I anticipate that life will provide me with security and stability across all areas.
5. **Remembrance -** I aim to make a lasting impact on others, so they remember me with affection.
6. **Fulfilment -** I seek contentment and satisfaction with my achievements.
7. **Perseverance -** I expect to persist in pursuing my goals despite any obstacles.

|| ॐ ||

Vijay Jain

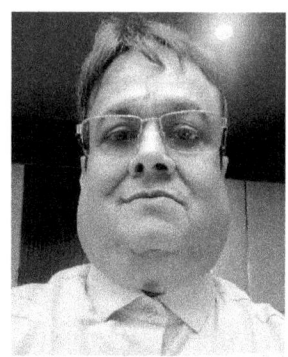

Author's Name	:	Vijay Jain
Qualification	:	B.Sc.
Current Profession	:	Astrologer and Vastu Consultant
Age	:	58 Years
E-mail ID	:	**vijayjain731@gmail.com**
City/ Country	:	**Kolkata, India**

Vijay Jain is a distinguished Astrologer, Vastu Expert, Graphologist and Pyramid Vastu Expert. Renowned for his profound knowledge and expertise, he has been honored with the prestigious Best Vastu Expert Award by the Economic Times and Dr. Jiten Bhatt, the esteemed founder of Pyramid Vastu. With a passion for enhancing lives through ancient wisdom and modern insights, Vijay Jain has dedicated himself to serving communities across the nation. His holistic approach and commitment to excellence have made him a trusted name in the field, empowering individuals and organizations to harness positive energies and achieve their fullest potential.

Vijay has the below LEEs of life :

Learning :

My learnings of life that can guide personal growth and fulfillment:

1. **Embrace Change :** Life is constantly changing, and resisting it only brings discomfort. Learn to adapt and flow with change, as it is the essence of growth. Each new phase brings new lessons and opportunities.
2. **Practice Gratitude :** Appreciating what you have, instead of focusing on what's missing, brings inner peace and joy. Gratitude shifts your mindset and attracts more positivity into your life.

3. **Live with Purpose :** A meaningful life is driven by purpose. Whether it's personal goals, contributing to society, or nurturing relationships, having a clear sense of purpose helps you stay motivated and focused on what truly matters.
4. **Forgive and Let Go :** Holding onto grudges or past pains only weighs you down. Forgiveness is a gift to yourself, freeing you from emotional burdens and allowing space for healing and growth.
5. **Self-Care is Essential :** You can't pour from an empty cup. Taking care of your physical, mental, and emotional well-being is crucial for your overall happiness and the ability to support others effectively.
6. **Failure is Part of Success :** Failure teaches resilience, patience, and valuable lessons. Embrace mistakes as opportunities for learning and growth. Every setback brings you closer to success if you approach it with the right mindset.
7. **Nurture Relationships :** Life is more meaningful when shared with others. Building strong, supportive relationships with family, friends, and colleagues fosters love, trust, and a sense of belonging.

These learnings shape how we navigate the complexities of life, helping us grow into more balanced, compassionate, and purposeful individuals.

Earning :

Seven important "earning" of life that go beyond material wealth, focusing on the deeper, more meaningful gains that truly enrich our lives:

1. **Self-Respect :** Earning respect from yourself by staying true to your values, principles, and maintaining integrity. When you respect yourself, you build a strong foundation for confidence and personal growth.
2. **Trust and Loyalty :** Trust is one of the most valuable things you can earn from others. Through honesty, consistency, and dependability, you gain the loyalty of friends, family, and colleagues.
3. **Love and Compassion :** Love isn't just given; it's earned through genuine care, kindness, and compassion towards others. Earning the love of people around you brings deeper, more fulfilling relationships.
4. **Wisdom :** Wisdom is earned through experience, reflection, and learning from both successes and failures. It's about understanding life's lessons and using them to make better decisions.
5. **Peace of Mind :** Earning peace of mind comes from living a life aligned with your values, resolving conflicts, letting go of negativity, and embracing a sense of contentment.
6. **Gratitude and Humility :** When you appreciate life's blessings, small or large, and remain humble in both success and failure, you earn inner satisfaction and the respect of others.
7. **Legacy and Impact :** The impact you leave behind—whether through kindness, teaching, mentorship, or contributions to your community—is an invaluable earning. A lasting legacy is built by positively influencing others and making the world a better place.

These are the true earnings of life that contribute to long-lasting fulfillment and a meaningful existence.

Expectation :

My seven expectations of life that can guide individuals toward growth, fulfillment, and a balanced approach to living:

1. **1. Expect Growth Through Challenges :** Life will present obstacles, but every challenge is an opportunity for personal growth. Expect to learn from difficulties and become stronger through resilience.

2. **Expect Imperfection :** Life isn't perfect, and neither are we. Expect mistakes, setbacks, and failures along the way, but view them as natural parts of the journey toward improvement.

3. **Expect Change :** Change is the only constant in life. Expect circumstances, people, and environments to evolve. Embracing this helps you stay adaptable and open to new opportunities.

4. **Expect Effort for Success :** Success in any area of life—personal, professional, or spiritual—requires consistent effort. Expect to work hard, remain disciplined, and stay committed to your goals.

5. **Expect Respect and Kindness :** It's reasonable to expect respect and kindness from others, as long as you also give the same in return. Mutual respect is key to healthy relationships and interactions.

6. **Expect Uncertainty :** Life is unpredictable. Expect moments of uncertainty and the unknown. Instead of fearing it, accept that uncertainty can lead to new experiences and growth.

7. **Expect Joy in Simple Things :** Expect happiness from the little moments—whether it's a sunrise, a smile, or a kind gesture. Life's true joys are often found in simplicity, not extravagance.

These expectations help maintain a balanced perspective, allowing for both acceptance of life's unpredictability and striving for personal achievement.

|| ॐ ||

Vijayshri Panchikal

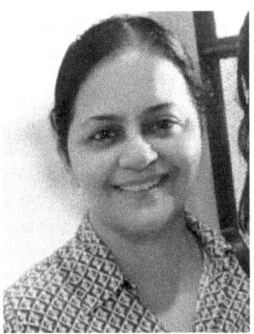

Author's Name	:	Vijayshri Panchikal
Qualification	:	Graduate
Current Profession	:	Counselor/ Therapist
Age	:	52 years
E-mail ID	:	**viji.panchikal@gmail.com**
City/ Country	:	**Bangalore, India**

Vijayshri Panchikal is a certified counsellor and founder of The Wisteria Centre, an emotional and mental wellbeing space, and the beacon, a career and college counselling venture in association with Proventus India. She brings years of rich experience and training in various other therapeutic modalities to this space. She is certified in Art therapist, a Therapeutic Dance in Education practitioner, an EFT Practitioner and is trained in NLP and Gestalt.

Vijayshri is an amateur artist and has held exhibitions successfully. She is also a published author.

Vijayshri has the below LEEs of life :

Learning :

1. To keep the curiosity alive and keep discovering oneself through learning new skill sets.
2. To keep training towards one's goals that are relevant to our interest.
3. To continuously expand one's horizons by never limiting ourselves to only what we think we can do or achieve.
4. Gain as much experience as possible in the areas of our specialization and make note of constructive feedback.

5. Look for opportunities to further your learning and growth holistically.

6. Incorporating daily wellbeing practices that will nurture your body, mind and soul.

7. Keep introspecting and reflecting on your inward and outward journey and how it has impacted your life and the life of those around you.

Earning :

1. Be open to explore different career paths or choices that align with your individual values, goals and dreams.

2. Qualifications, certifications and training are important, so educate yourself accordingly.

3. Start building up experience by applying what you learn in order to advance your career/ profession for better satisfaction and brighter prospects.

4. Track your progress.

5. Pursue opportunities that highlight your expertise and showcase your contributions and talent.

6. Being conscious about maintaining a healthy work-life balance.

7. Reflect on your work and how it can continue to have a positive impact on those around you.

Expectation :

1. Keep an open mind and have realistic expectations about what it is that you want to achieve.

2. Keep tracking advancements in your area of work and tweak your expectations accordingly.

3. Be prepared for good and bad, successes and setbacks, criticism and praise and course correct as needed.

4. Continuous and consistent effort to reach our goals.

5. Balancing our professional expectations and personal life needs at all times.

6. The legacy you want to leave behind.

7. No expectation is an essential expectation

|| ॐ ||

Viji S

Author's Name	:	Viji S
Qualification	:	M.A., M.Phil., B.L.I.S.
Current Profession	:	Guest Lecturer
Age	:	36 years
E-mail ID	:	…
City/ Country	:	**Tamil Nadu, India**

Viji is a budding author and an educator. She is always curious to learn new things. She is a good listener, detailed-oriented person, sel-motivated, hardworking person with positive attitude towards her life and career. During her leisure time she enjoys listening to music, reading and drawing.

Expect the least, and do your best to earn happiness and be the lesson for others to learn to earn happiness without expectation. I strongly believe that **"Seven Lee of Life"** book is put together to elivate everyone to ace in life. My **LEEs** of life are as under

Learning :

1. Learning makes humans wise – which
2. Earns respect twice;
3. Adept at acquiring emerging concepts – which
4. Rejuvenates spirits to be high;
5. No age limit and limitations for learning – which
6. Earnestly caters happiness and hopes brightens around;
7. Realise learning makes humans alive.

Earning :

1. Earn! Earn! Earn!
2. Adore to earn and give love,
3. Recognise to earn sound health is vital,
4. Never fail to earn trust,

5. Ignite earning self confidence in life,
6. Nothing should stop you from earning success,
7. Get out of your way to earn peaceful life.

Expectation :
1. Expectation on others only will hurt you, not within you;
2. Xanadu and be
3. Positive in
4. Expecting to be better you tomorrow for which,
5. Clarify your role in life and
6. Trust you can reach your expectation then
7. Success is yours forever.

|| ॐ ||

Vinieta

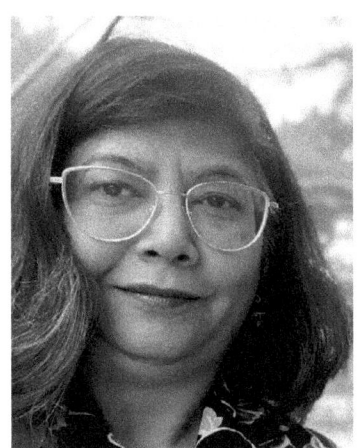

Author's Name	:	Vinieta
Qualification	:	B.E. (Electrical), M.B.A
Current Profession	:	Information Technology Services
Age	:	56 years
E-mail ID	:	**vinieta00@gmail.com**
City/ Country	:	**Gurugram, India**

Vinieta is a Meditation Teacher associated with Ananda Sangha and is a disciple of Paramhansa Yogananda, author of Autobiography of a Yogi. She has been sharing her guru's teachings through offline/online classes in Hindi and English. She is a Certified Ananda Yoga Teacher.

She is an engineer, currently working in the field of Information Technology in a reputed Petroleum sector Consultancy. She did her M.B.A. from University of Ljubljana, Slovenia. An avid reader and enthusiast traveler who has visited number of European, African and Asian countries and various cities in India.

She loves playing Badminton, Carrom and Chess and has been representing her company in Carrom and Badminton in various tournaments.

She has been working towards upliftment of and spreading awareness amongst the downtrodden.

Writing poetry is her passion along with chanting spiritual chants - mainly of Paramhansa Yogananda and Swami Kriyananda, direct disciple of Yogananda and founder of Ananda.

Anthology on *Seven LEE of Life* is collection of thoughts, opinions and interesting as well as diverse perspectives put together at one place in this book. It gives the learnings a person has collected while travelling on the journey of life; the earnings not material, but valuable yet invisible accomplishments of the person that define the personality of the author.

This series gives an insight to what really matters to a person in the end. The reader is bound to relate to one or more LEE because experiences are different yet similar as one faces challenges only as learning or a blessing. Inspiring, interesting and thought-provoking LEE make for a must read for all times and ages.

From LEE we can infer Learnings, Earnings and Expectations of life.

Learning :

1. **Doer:** God is the doer and we are just channels of his work.
2. **Blessings:** Life consists of only two things – Learnings and blessings
3. **Surrender:** Once we surrender to the Divine, Universe creatively places everything in a win-win scenario, beyond expectations.
4. **Patience:** Right things happen only at the right time, never before and never after.
5. **Expectation:** Expectation leads to disappointment so do anything and everything without thinking about the result.
6. **Repetitiveness:** Never make the same mistake twice.
7. **Forgiveness:** By forgiving and forgetting, one becomes light and free of burden and shackles of ego.

Earning :

1. **Goodwill:** Have a good rapport with all because of which people give their time and support.
2. **Respect:** People acknowledge and give respect not because of any position but the positivity they experience while interacting.
3. **Voice:** Sweetness in voice through chanting with harmonium.
4. **Child:** A child who has grown up into a good human being and a supportive family.
5. **Awareness:** Heightened awareness of surroundings, happenings and Divine guidance.
6. **Education:** Good education with good communication skills and abundance around.
7. **Telepathy:** Whenever someone is in thoughts a lot, there is a call or a message from that person.

Expectation:

1. **Medium:** Desire to be a good channel for spreading Guru's teachings and contribute in making this world a better place to live.
2. **Guidance:** I will think and act willingly, but only guided by thou, my Guru.

3. **Freedom:** To be able to put in energy to be free of every attachment.

4. **Contentment:** I will get whatever I need, at the time I need it.

5. **Purpose-fulfillment:** To be able to achieve the soul purpose.

6. **Support:** Support and help in creating an environment where everyone shares and helps each other.

7. **Expectation:** Expect not to expect my share as everything in the Universe is mine.

|| ॐ ||

Vishal Sachdev

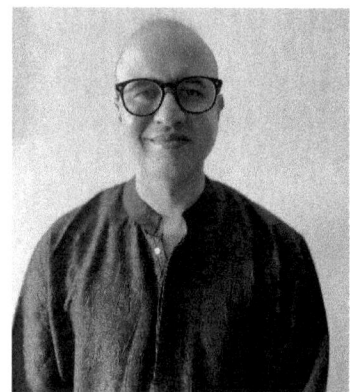

Author's Name	:	Vishal Sachdev
Qualification	:	Post Graduate in Personnel Management
Current Profession	:	HR Consultant, Yoga Trainer, Numerologist & Tarot Card reader
Age	:	49 years
E-mail ID	:	**vishals65@hotmail.com**
City/ Country	:	**Bangalore, India**

Vishal Sachdev is HR Professional turned Numerologist & Tarot Card Reader.

He has over two decades of experience in the IT industry handling Talent Acquisition. He is a post graduate in personnel management & business administration. He has worked with several MNC s like HPE, SAP, IBM etc.

Vishal is a certified Numerologist & Tarot Card reader. Qualified in Vaastu Shastra & is a qualified practicing Yoga Trainer.

The word Anthology came from the 17th century Greek word anthologia for "flower gathering" or collecting. An anthology means collaboration with a group of people and also means numerous energies are backing a specific project.

'Seven LEE of Life' is an interesting topic giving different perspectives on the topic within an anthology. Number 7 plays a significant role in our life it is regarded as mysterious & spiritual number. In the old Testament, God rested on the seventh day after creating the world in six days.The number seven believes in seeing beyond the face and understanding the hidden truth. Nature represents seven colours in the rainbow, seven wonders of the world & seven seas. As an early prime number in the series of positive integers, the number seven in religion, mythology, superstition & philosophy.

The seven chakras control energies in a human body. Having inspired by this following an attempt to decipher the seven LEE of life. I have made an attempt to use quotes which help understand Life, Earning and Expectation in a better manner.

I have chosen these quotes since I do see strong resonance with life and these are quotes that can be best applied in our life. The beauty with quotes are that in just a few words the essence of a life concept is easy to present & comprehend.

This anthology gives us an opportunity with so many different perspectives.... My LEEs are as under:

Learning:

1. Never stop learning since life doesn't stop teaching.
2. The capacity to learn is a gift, the ability to learn is a skill, the willingness to learn is a choice.
3. A happy life is one spent in learning earning & yearning.
4. Focus on Learning, Not Earning, Learning Always happens in Present While Earning Always are in Future
5. Knowledge is a treasure, but practice is the key to it
6. Knowledge is like a garden if its not cultivated it can't be harvested
7. An investment in learning always pays the best Interest

Earning:

1. Self-belief & Hard work will always earn you success
2. The key to earning more is: To Keep your learning ahead of your Earning
3. If you really want to earn, earn people in life, Not money
4. Real wealth is not about money, but real wealth is about Freedom
5. Earning a lot of money is not the key to prosperity; How you handle it is.
6. Its not how much you earn, its how much you keep
7. Money is not everything but everything needs money

Expectation:

1. Expect nothing and you will never be disappointed
2. If you want to be happy have zero expectations of others
3. Peace begins when expectation ends.
4. Hope but never expect, Look forward but never wait
5. Some times we create our own heartbreaks through expectations

6. Expect more from yourself and less from others
7. Don't blame people for disappointing you, blame yourself for expecting too much from them

॥ ॐ ॥

Blurb

Dive into the profound depths of **'Seven LEE of Life'**, an extraordinary anthology featuring the insights and perspectives of 108 unique co-authors, where they share their unique perspectives on the essence of life through the lenses of ***'Learning, Earning and Expectation'***. Each contributor distils their insights into seven compelling points, creating the pillars of wisdom and inspiration. This book is more than a collection of thoughts; it's an ocean of ideas that explores the interplay of growth, financial prosperity and future aspirations on personal and professional level. This anthology can be a holistic view through diverse voices and varied experiences or a deeper understanding of your own path.

The book promises to be a valuable companion, embark on a transformative journey and uncover the seven keys on each point to a fulfilling life, shaped by the collective wisdom of 108 esteemed authors. Whether you're seeking motivation, guidance or a fresh outlook, **'Seven LEE of Life'** offers a treasure trove of reflections to navigate the journey of life.

|| ॐ ||

Gratitude to Readers

Dear Readers,

With every word crafted in *Seven LEE of Life,* we aimed to build a bridge of shared experiences and insights and it's your open hearts that bring this vision to life. You are the ones who complete this journey, transforming thoughts into meaning and opinion into shared wisdom. Together with Rainu Mangtani and Abhishaik Chitraans, profoundly grateful for your time, trust and openness as you walk this path of **Learning, Earning** and **Expectation** with us.

Your support not only honors our efforts, but uplifts each of the 108 voices that contributed to these pages. Thank you for making this anthology a part of your world; may it add value to yours as it has to ours.

With deep gratitude and respect,

Rainu Mangtani
Abhishaik Chitraans
(ईष्ट कृपा एवं गुरु आशीष)

॥ ॐ ॥

Kindly Connect with Us and share your Feedbacks/ Reviews

✉ ankakshrmiracless@gmail.com

Full Name :

Nick/ Popular Name :

Name of Spouse :

Date of Birth :   Date of Marriage :

Profession :

WhatsApp Number :   Social Media handle :

Email ID :

City/ Country :   Pincode:

Reviews/ Feedback :

Thanks for your Time & Efforts

॥ ॐ ॥

List of Books

Books written by Abhishaik Chitraans:

1. **Sex**: A Complex Intersection of Physical Need and Mental Well-being
2. **Life**: A Dance of Light and Shadow
3. **The God's Tender**: Love & Care
4. **Mobile Addiction:** 21 Simple Techniques to Remove or Reduce Mobile Addiction in Children/ Students and Adults
5. **P³**: The Triple Power of Alphabet–P (Proud, Pain, Prayer)

Books written by Rainu Mangtani:

1. **The Height of Life in 24 Rains**: An Inspirational Auto Biography
2. **Today's Corporate World**: A Robotic Mechanism of Youth
3. **Ladder of Success**: Best 15 Ways to Achieve Your Goals

i) **Deep Secrets of Name :** A comprehensive book on advanced Name Numerology based on Chaldean System & an extensive research based on real life case studies. The best book on Name Numerology by 3 eminent Indian authors in Google search, launched at Pragati Maidan, New Delhi in World Book Fair 2024.

Mr. Abhishaik Chitraans is as main Author/ Guide of the book with the two renowned authors and research scholars of Numerology namely Mrs. Rainu Mangtani (Numerologist & Graphologist) and Mrs. Jyotsnaa G Bansal (Astro-Numerologist).

ii) **Women Empowerment and Economic Developments :** An anthology/ articles collection of 51 Co-Authors, lunched on occasion of International Women's Day and Mahashivratri, 08th March, 2024 with online presence of Padma Shri recipient Smt. Gulabo Sapera ji, a legendary folk artist.

|| ॐ ||

शब्दों का समंदर है यह,

बस डूबकर पढ़ते जाना है।

इंतजार करो किताब का अगली,

हमें काफिला बड़ा बनाना है।।

रेनू – अभिषेक

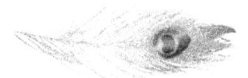

E-mail : ankakshrmiracless@gmail.com
Whatsapp # +91-9368746306

www.ingramcontent.com/pod-product-compliance
Lightning Source LLC
LaVergne TN
LVHW070538070526
838199LV00076B/6802